Complications of Temporomandibular Joint Surgery

Gary F. Bouloux
Editor

Complications of Temporomandibular Joint Surgery

Springer

Editor
Gary F. Bouloux
Emory University School of Medicine
Department of Surgery Emory University
School of Medicine
Atlanta, Georgia
USA

ISBN 978-3-319-51239-6 ISBN 978-3-319-51241-9 (eBook)
DOI 10.1007/978-3-319-51241-9

Library of Congress Control Number: 2017940887

Printed on acid-free paper

This Springer imprint is published by Springer Nature
The registered company is Springer International Publishing AG
The registered company address is: Gewerbestrasse 11, 6330 Cham, Switzerland

Foreword

Surgeons and patients alike fear complications. No one expects them, but unfortunately they still occur even when the surgeon has taken every reasonable precaution to prevent them and when the patient is the ideal candidate for the procedure.

Surgical complications as a fact of clinical life vary in frequency based, to a great extent, on the degree of difficulty of the operative procedure. The more complicated the procedure, the more likely complications will arise. Surgery of the temporomandibular joint (TMJ) is widely accepted as one of the most complicated operations one can perform. The anatomy of the TMJ and close proximity of vital structures such as the facial nerve, ear canal, brain, and sizable vessels are major reasons for the high degree of difficulty with TMJ surgery. In addition, the ginglymoarthrodial nature of the joint and its effects on the occlusion and facial form increase the surgical challenge. The relatively small size of the joint also requires surgical finesse. Finally, many patients requiring TMJ surgery suffer severe chronic pain and, in some cases, previous complications of TMJ procedures that makes it difficult to achieve ideal outcomes.

Complications of Temporomandibular Joint Surgery is a welcome addition to the surgical literature. Its chapters cover all of the major complications of TMJ surgery. The multi-author nature of the book brings the reader information and analysis from an impressive Who's Who of widely recognized experts in the field of TMJ surgery. The book offers the reader not only the latest evidence-based guidelines for the management of complications but also, as importantly, guidance on how to lessen the chances of having complications occur.

Complications of Temporomandibular Joint Surgery will be required reading for all residents who are training to perform TMJ surgery, as well as for all surgeons who have TMJ surgery as a part of their surgical practice. As a surgeon who absolutely hates complications, I am thankful that many very busy surgical colleagues took the time and effort to share their extensive knowledge and expertise with the world.

James Hupp DMD, MD, JD
Editor in Chief, Journal of Oral and Maxillofacial Surgery
Fairfield Glade, Tennessee, USA

Contents

1 Failure to Make the Correct Diagnosis: Part I – A Neurologist's Perspective

Andrew Guidry and Gregory J. Esper

1.1 Introduction

A basic knowledge of headache is important in treating the pre- and postoperative temporomandibular joint (TMJ) surgical patient. Understanding the epidemiological characteristics of headaches, headache types, treatments of headache, and current clinical data will help practitioners make the correct diagnosis initially. This will allow the surgeon to better identify a good surgical candidate as well as recognize other sources of head pain requiring diagnosis and treatment. A directed history and pertinent physical examination combined with an algorithmic approach will lead to the correct diagnosis and treatment of most headaches.

1.2 Epidemiology

According to the World Health Organization in 2012, 50–75% of the global adult population had at least one headache in the last year [1]. One such headache disorder is headache attributed to temporomandibular disorder (TMD), which is classified as a secondary headache caused by a disorder involving structures in the temporomandibular region [2].

Temporomandibular joint dysfunction remains common with approximately 75% of the US population having at least one sign or symptom of TMD during their lifetime [3]. Additionally the prevalence of TMD is estimated to be 46.1% with at

A. Guidry, MD (✉)
Department of Neurology, The Sandra and Malcolm Berman Brain and Spine Institute, Baltimore, MD, USA
e-mail: aguidry@lifebridgehealth.org

G.J. Esper, MD, MBA
Emory University School of Medicine, Atlanta, GA, USA
e-mail: gesper@emory.edu

G.F. Bouloux (ed.), *Complications of Temporomandibular Joint Surgery*,
DOI 10.1007/978-3-319-51241-9_1

least 10% of the population having a painful TMJ [3–5]. The prevalence of TMD is also higher in the headache population than in the general population [6]. When considering individuals diagnosed with a headache disorder, there is a 56.1% prevalence of concomitant TMD [6]. Conversely, patients diagnosed with TMD are also very likely to report headaches with an incidence that approaches 80% [7]. Despite the strong association between TMD and headache, it behooves the surgeon to accurately diagnose the etiology of headache prior to considering any treatment for TMD.

1.3 Pathophysiology

As a part of the process of diagnosing and treating headache, it is important for the surgeon to identify conditions causing headaches that can be serious. Signs and symptoms of a potentially serious condition may include the sudden onset of the "worst headache of life", fever, meningismus, chronic and worsening holocephalic head pain over weeks to months, worsening vision changes that do not resolve, focal neurologic findings, severe unilateral head pain in an elderly person with tenderness, jaw claudication, and vision changes and headaches that frequently wake the patient from sleep. If any of these findings are present, neurology consultation and imaging should be performed early.

In order to differentiate TMD from other headache types, the surgeon must be able to recognize and diagnose the following headache types:

- Migraine
- Tension-type headache
- Chronic daily headache
- Trigeminal neuralgia
- Persistent idiopathic facial pain
- Cluster headache
- Trigeminal autonomic cephalalgia
- Giant cell arteritis
- Neoplasm
- Cervicogenic headache
- Temporomandibular disorder headache

1.3.1 Migraine

The prevalence of migraine and tension-type headache (TTH) is higher in the TMD population [6]. For this reason, understanding both of these headache types is necessary. The typical presentation of migraine is a severely intense unilateral headache with a throbbing sensation with associated photophobia, phonophobia, and nausea. If the patient had a sensory or visual complaint associated with this type of headache, then the patient may have migraine with aura. Patients may give a description of having to go rest in a dark room for several hours and stop their daily activities with the onset of a migraine (Box 1.1).

Box 1.1: Migraine Without Aura [2]

A. At least five attacks fulfilling criteria B–D
B. Headache attacks lasting 4–72 hours (untreated or unsuccessfully treated)
C. Headache has at least two of the following four characteristics:
   1. Unilateral location
   2. Pulsating quality
   3. Moderate or severe pain intensity
   4. Aggravation by or causing avoidance of routine physical activity (e.g., walking or climbing stairs)
D. During headache at least one of the following:
   1. Nausea and/or vomiting
   2. Photophobia and phonophobia
E. Not better accounted for by another ICHD-3 diagnosis

Although variations do occur, the patient may recall that they once had similar headaches in their teenage years. Migraine may also resolve for an extended period of time only to return later in life. Other patients may already have a diagnosis of migraine that tends to occur only once or twice a year but report that the same headache is now more frequent. Migraine frequency may change for multiple reasons including changes in stress, sleep, mood, and hormonal fluctuations. Migraine quality, laterality, and associated symptoms such as photophobia and nausea may also change over time. The use of abortive and prophylactic medications to manage migraine should be accomplished through referral to a primary care physician or neurologist.

1.3.2 Tension-Type Headache (TTH)

The typical presentation of TTH is a mild bilateral headache with a pressure or aching sensation that may or may not have photophobia or phonophobia. Less than ten headaches of this type per month suggests the diagnosis of infrequent episodic TTH, while more than ten headaches per month suggests frequent episodic TTH.

Pericranial tenderness or myofascial pain is pain that occurs over any portion of the cranium that is the result of trigger points in the muscle, fascia, or tendons that produce local or referred pain [4]. Therefore, if a patient meets the criteria for TTH and has pain to palpation over the area of the headache (typically temporal regions), the patient has TTH with pericranial pain rather than the classic myofascial pain seen in a proportion of TMD patients. Treatment is primarily directed at reducing trigger point sensitivity.

Tension-type headache is one of the most common headache syndromes, but infrequently comes to the attention of healthcare professionals because it tends to respond well to nonprescription medications. Sleep hygiene, hydration, adequate nutrition, and stress management are important lifestyle factors that must be addressed in patients with TTH. These factors are important to manage in all headache types as they are common headache triggers. Appropriate non-pharmacologic interventions should be a mainstay of treatment for patients with frequent episodic TTH (Box 1.2).

Box 1.2: Infrequent Episodic Tension-Type Headache [2]

A. At least ten episodes of headache occurring on <1 day per month on average (<12 days per year) and fulfilling criteria B–D
B. Lasting from 30 minutes to 7 days
C. At least two of the following four characteristics:
   1. Bilateral location
   2. Pressing or tightening (non-pulsating) quality
   3. Mild or moderate intensity
   4. Not aggravated by routine physical activity such as walking or climbing stairs
D. Both of the following:
   1. No nausea or vomiting
   2. No more than one of photophobia or phonophobia
E. Not better accounted for by another ICHD-3 diagnosis

1.3.3 Chronic Daily Headache

Most headache types can evolve into chronic daily headache (CDH). If patients with migraines or TTH stated that headaches occurred daily, then that meets the definition of chronic daily headache. There is no separate category for CDH based on the third edition of the International Classification of Headache Disorders. Many CDHs are the result of failure to treat other aspects of a patient's headache rather than a new type of headache for the patient. In addition to the lifestyle triggers mentioned previously, medication overuse and depression can be factors in the evolution of CDH.

While infrequent use of nonsteroidal anti-inflammatories, acetaminophen, and narcotics can benefit CDH, frequent use can create complex physiological changes such as receptor downregulation resulting in CDH. Medication withdrawal can exacerbate the pain. Chronic daily headache is often related to medication overuse, and a patient must cease all abortive medications for an extended period of time (e.g. 2 months) before CDH not related to medication overuse can be diagnosed.

Sleep is very important to headache management, and a basic sleep questionnaire should be included in taking a focused headache history. These questions should address quantity and quality of sleep in addition to snoring. Snoring may be a sign of obstructive sleep apnea, which is a common cause of chronic daily headache. Such headaches are often worse in the morning and are alleviated during the day, as the vasodilatory effects of high carbon dioxide wear off with wakeful ventilation. If there is no concern for sleep apnea, appropriate sleep hygiene will benefit patients. Avoiding meals before bedtime, avoiding bright lights before sleep, sleeping at the same time each night to achieve between six and nine hours of sleep per night, and sleeping in the same setting are all behavioral changes that will improve sleep hygiene.

1.3.4 Trigeminal Neuralgia

Trigeminal neuralgia has some similarities with TMD due to the trigeminal nerve and its facial sensory distribution and motor activity on the muscles of mastication [11]. The typical presentation of trigeminal neuralgia is a severe sharp or electrical shooting pain that lasts for a few seconds to two minutes on one side of the face in one of the distributions of the trigeminal nerve. With respect to the divisions of the trigeminal nerve and the frequency of involvement, V2 > V3 > V1. Rare bilateral cases have also been reported. The pain is typically provoked by chewing or pressure on the affected area that is innervated by the trigeminal nerve. Diurnal variation is often present with few nocturnal symptoms.

The initial treatment for trigeminal neuralgia is with antiepileptic medications, such as carbamazepine, gabapentin, and lamotrigine. Other more aggressive therapies can be used if medications are ineffective including radiofrequency ablation and microvascular decompression of the trigeminal nerve.

There is a variation of trigeminal neuralgia that has been termed as pre-trigeminal neuralgia. This term is rarely used today but was introduced in 1980 for an already-known phenomenon related to trigeminal neuralgia that was later summarized in an article in 1990 [12]. The definition for pre-trigeminal neuralgia is a nonspecific continuous dull pain in the region of the upper or lower jaw that is often mistaken for sinus or dental pain where the pain becomes the typical trigeminal neuralgia pain in the distribution of the trigeminal nerve anywhere from a few days to several years later after the onset of the dull pain. This pain responds to the same therapies used for trigeminal neuralgia (Box 1.3).

Box 1.3: Trigeminal Neuralgia [2]

A. At least three attacks of unilateral facial pain fulfilling criteria B and C
B. Occurring in one or more divisions of the trigeminal nerve, with no radiation beyond the trigeminal distribution
C. Pain has at least three of the following four characteristics:
   1. Recurring in paroxysmal attacks lasting from a fraction of a second to 2 minutes
   2. Severe intensity
   3. Electric shock-like, shooting, stabbing, or sharp in quality
   4. Precipitated by innocuous stimuli to the affected side of the face
D. No clinically evident neurological deficit
E. Not better accounted for by another ICHD-3 diagnosis

1.3.5 Persistent Idiopathic Facial Pain

Persistent idiopathic facial pain (PIFP) typically presents as a dull, daily continuous pain that has no localizing features and does not follow the distribution of a cranial nerve and is not related to an identifiable source of dental pain. The historical term atypical facial pain (AFP) has been replaced with PIFP. The pain associated with PIFP may also be sharp. The diagnosis of PIFP should be reserved for cases where all other causes of facial pain have been eliminated. In addition, PIFP has an association with other pain syndromes including postsurgical facial pain, trigeminal neuralgia, atypical odontalgia, and psychiatric comorbidities [2]. As previously mentioned, PIFP may precede typical trigeminal neuralgia under the definition of pre-trigeminal neuralgia. Studies have shown that PIFP can coexist with trigeminal neuralgia in up to 42% of patients as the dull pain persists even after the onset of typical trigeminal neuralgia and should be treated as a separate pain syndrome [13]. Treatment is conservative management, and if there is an association with trigeminal neuralgia, pharmacological therapies for trigeminal neuralgia may be tried. Other options besides surgery should be considered as surgery usually worsens the pain in PIFP (Box 1.4).

Box 1.4: Persistent Idiopathic Facial Pain [2]

A. Facial and/or oral pain fulfilling criteria B and C
B. Recurring daily for >2 hours per day for >3 months
C. Pain has both of the following characteristics:
   1. Poorly localized and not following the distribution of a peripheral nerve
   2. Dull, aching, or nagging quality
D. Clinical neurological examination is normal
E. A dental cause has been excluded by appropriate investigations
F. Not better accounted for by another ICHD-3 diagnosis

1.3.6 Cluster Headache

Cluster headache symptoms are rarely confused for TMD although it remains important to identify these as they are treatable. Most forms of cluster headache will have symptomatic orbital or ocular involvement, and patients will give a description of an episodic pattern to the headache as well as a sensation of restlessness. The condition is more common in males and often associated with rhinorrhea, epiphora, and flushing of the skin.

The primary treatment for cluster headache is the administration of oxygen. If oxygen is unsuccessful, many of the medications used to treat migraine can be considered as well as surgical sympathectomy (Box 1.5).

Box 1.5: Cluster Headache [2]

A. At least five attacks fulfilling criteria B–D
B. Severe or very severe unilateral orbital, supraorbital, and/or temporal pain lasting 15–180 minutes (when untreated)
C. Either or both of the following:
   1. At least one of the following symptoms or signs, ipsilateral to the headache:
      (a) Conjunctival injection and/or lacrimation
      (b) Nasal congestion and/or rhinorrhea
      (c) Eyelid edema
      (d) Forehead and facial sweating
      (e) Forehead and facial flushing
      (f) Sensation of fullness in the ear
      (g) Miosis and/or ptosis
   2. A sense of restlessness or agitation
D. Attacks have a frequency between one every other day and eight per day for more than half of the time when the disorder is active
E. Not better accounted for by another ICHD-3 diagnosis

1.3.7 Trigeminal Autonomic Cephalalgia

The trigeminal autonomic cephalalgia (TAC) headaches are similar to cluster headache but differ with respect to the duration and frequency of symptoms. They likely share a similar pathophysiology. Each painful episode tends to be of shorter duration although the frequency of episodes is higher. The sensation of restlessness or agitation can occur in both TACs and cluster headaches. The primary differences between TACs and cluster headache are the increased frequency of painful episodes with TAC and the fact that TAC can often be treated with indomethacin. Additionally the ability to prevent an episode with indomethacin is one of the diagnostic criteria for TAC headaches [2]. Trigeminal autonomic cephalalgia can be further divided into paroxysmal hemicrania and hemicrania continua, the difference related to the duration of painful episodes and periods or remission.

1.3.8 Giant Cell Arteritis

Failure to recognize and treat giant cell arteritis (GCA) can lead to serious and permanent consequences. New onset headache without a prior headache history should alert the surgeon to the potential for GCA. Giant cell arteritis, an inflammatory condition of the cranial arteries, should be considered in any patient over the age of 50 with a new type of headache [3]. If untreated, giant cell arteritis can lead to permanent vision loss. Serum erythrocyte sedimentation rate and C-reactive protein should be ordered and are typically abnormally high. If laboratory workup is equivocal or unclear and the suspicion remains high for giant cell arteritis, then a temporal artery biopsy should be pursued. The initiation of treatment for giant cell arteritis should not be delayed, and high-dose corticosteroids should be started immediately if there is suspicion for this disease [3] (Box 1.6).

Box 1.6: Giant Cell Arteritis [2]

A. Any new headache fulfilling criterion C
B. Giant cell arteritis (GCA) has been diagnosed
C. Evidence of causation demonstrated by at least two of the following:
   1. Headache has developed in close temporal relation to other symptoms and/or clinical or biological signs of onset of GCA or has led to the diagnosis of GCA
   2. Either or both of the following:
      (a) Headache has significantly worsened in parallel with worsening of GCA
      (b) Headache has significantly improved or resolved within 3 days of high-dose steroid treatment
   3. Headache is associated with scalp tenderness and/or jaw claudication
D. Not better accounted for by another ICHD-3 diagnosis

1.3.9 Neoplasm

Neoplasm should always be considered as a potential cause in new onset headache that does not fit the classic clinical presentations of migraine, cluster headache, and other well-defined headache syndromes. Headaches from neoplasm are nonspecific and can present with a variety of symptoms. Classic symptoms from an intracranial mass include subacute to chronic progressive pain minimally relieved with medications, pain worse with Valsalva maneuvers or laying down, and neurological deficits including vision changes and paresthesias that are more chronic than those occurring with aura. An MRI with and without contrast is sufficient to make the diagnosis.

1.3.10 Cervicogenic Headache

Cervicogenic headache is a headache caused by the cervical spine and its components including fascia, muscles, and nerves [2]. Headache that starts in the back of the head or is associated with neck pain may suggest cervicogenic headache.

The confluence of upper cervical afferent somatosensory neurons synapse in the spinal nucleus of the trigeminal nerve meaning that sensory input from the cervical region terminates in the trigeminal spinal nucleus as well as input from the trigeminal nerve itself [3, 10]. This synapse explains how pain from the cervical region may refer to the face [3, 10]. Cervicogenic headache will be further discussed in this chapter (Box 1.7).

Box 1.7: Cervicogenic Headache [2]

A. Any headache fulfilling criterion C
B. Clinical, laboratory, and/or imaging evidence of a disorder or lesion within the cervical spine or soft tissues of the neck, known to be able to cause headache
C. Evidence of causation demonstrated by at least two of the following:
   1. Headache has developed in temporal relation to the onset of the cervical disorder or appearance of the lesion
   2. Headache has significantly improved or resolved in parallel with improvement in or resolution of the cervical disorder or lesion
   3. Cervical range of motion is reduced and headache is made significantly worse by provocative maneuvers
   4. Headache is abolished following diagnostic blockade of a cervical structure or its nerve supply
D. Not better accounted for by another ICHD-3 diagnosis

1.3.11 Temporomandibular Disorder Headache

Temporomandibular joint dysfunction includes both myofascial pain dysfunction and pathology of the temporomandibular joint (TMJ) itself [5]. It can be challenging and difficult to differentiate pain emanating from the TMJ or from other structures in the temporomandibular region. In order to better identify TMD, the surgeon must obtain a thorough history and perform a focused physical examination. Factors and activities that increase or ameliorate pain are critical to making the correct diagnosis. Distinguishing intra-articular pain from myofascial pain and the multitude of other headache causes is essential. More than one disorder is often present further compounding the situation. Intra-articular TMJ pain is often worse when opening and closing the jaw and may or may not be associated with joint sounds and limited opening [3, 4, 10]. The presence of capsular tenderness and a positive Mahan test may further support the diagnosis. Tenderness to palpation over the muscles of mastication may also suggest myofascial pain. In reality multiple headache types can also present with a similar finding.

The first-line treatment for TMD is typically conservative management. For those patients who are refractory to conservative treatment, surgery is an option. Overall, studies suggest at least a 50% reduction in headache after TMJ surgery [14–16]. As a part of surgical therapy, the other aspects of conservative management remain crucial as all of those therapies need to be utilized after surgery. In particular, educating the patient on expected outcomes is important since not all patients have resolution of headache after surgery.

1.4 Case Scenarios

In this scenario, the patient provides sparse information, and the practitioner needs to know how to take a detailed headache history (Box 1.8).

Box 1.8: Headache History

When did the headache first start in life?

- How often does the headache occur?
- How long does the headache last?
- Where does the headache start?
- What is the quality of the headache pain? (sharp, throbbing, dull, aching, etc.)
- What triggers or worsens the headache?
- Does chewing severely worsen the headache?
- Prior headache history?
- How many hours of sleep a night?
- Is there fatigue on first awakening?
- Has anyone mentioned that the patient snores?

For these questions, the practitioner must know how to tease out accurate information from the patient. When patients present to the clinic in pain, most patients state that their entire head hurts. In addition, most activities including chewing will worsen any type of headache to some degree. Therefore, the practitioner needs to identify when the act of chewing is the primary action that exacerbates pain, which is the case in TMD (Cases 1.1 and 1.2).

Case 1.1: Scenario

A 35-year-old woman with no significant past medical history presents to clinic with an active headache. She states that the headache lasts several hours and more recently has started to cause her to miss work. When the headache is most intense, her whole head hurts, she has pain in her right ear, and she does not feel like eating. She says that over-the-counter medications provide minimal relief.

A. Migraine

She states that the headache first started about 2 years ago and happens one to two times a month. She states that once the headache starts, the headache lasts the entire day. The headache starts on the right side of her head and is a throbbing sensation. Poor sleep and stress are her triggers, but most nights she gets 8 hours of sleep, does not snore, and wakes up rested. She notices that bright lights and loud sounds worsen her headache but does not notice any sensory abnormalities. Although chewing worsens her headache some, she could eat if needed. She denies having headaches in the past.

Exam: No cranial nerve deficits and the rest of the neurological exam is normal. Mild pain to palpation over the right temporalis and no pain to palpation over the right TMJ.
Additional diagnostic studies needed: None
Diagnosis: Migraine without aura
Treatment: Migraine abortive pharmaceutical therapy and appropriate sleep hygiene

B. Tension-type headache

She states that the headache first started over the last year and happens one to two times a week. She states that most headaches start near the end of her work day and then last 2–3 hours, but she is able to complete any errands after work. Her headaches occur across her forehead into her temples. The pain is dull and pressure-like. Bright lights worsen her headache but she has no nausea and no problems with sound. She denies that pain radiates from her ear but states that the headache is worse on the right side at times. Often times, she skips meals and will sometimes complete her nightly errands and just go to sleep instead of eating dinner. Chewing on tough, solid foods can worsen the headache some but most foods and liquids do not cause issues. She has had similar headaches throughout most of her adult life but not at this frequency. She notes that she is not sleeping well by only getting 5–6 hours of sleep a night and that she started a new job over the last year. She does not snore but wakes up fatigued.

Exam: No cranial nerve deficits and the rest of the neurological exam is normal. Mild pressure sensation to palpation over the bilateral temporalis and no pain to palpation over the TMJs.
Additional diagnostic studies needed: None
Diagnosis: Infrequent episodic TTH
Treatment: Over-the-counter NSAID or acetaminophen abortive therapy and appropriate sleep hygiene

C. Trigeminal neuralgia

She states that the headache started over the last year and occur multiple times a week. She states that each episode starts with a severe sharp and stabbing pain in the right side of her face that is followed by a dull ache. She says that the sharp component lasts about a minute and that the dull ache can continue for 2–3 hours. She clarifies that the sharp sensation occurs mainly in her right cheek and inside of her mouth. Chewing, sleeping on the right side of her face, and cold water tend to cause her headache. Until the last year, she has never had this type of headache before. If the pain does not wake her up, she gets 8 hours of sleep a night, does not snore, and wakes up rested.

Exam: No cranial nerve deficits and the rest of the neurological exam is normal. Applied pressure to each TMJ does not elicit pain, but a glass of cold water induces her headache in the office.
Additional diagnostic studies needed: MRI/MRA brain
Diagnosis: Trigeminal neuralgia
Treatment: Daily carbamazepine

D. Cluster headache

She states that the headaches started over the last year and occurs multiple times a day for a few days and then she will go a few weeks without a headache. Each headache lasts 2 hours. The headache starts behind the right eye and radiates through the orbit and over her right temple, and she begins to feels pressure in her right ear. The headache is described as a severe stabbing pain. She denies any triggers for the headache, and she does not have photophobia and phonophobia. Chewing causes minimal discomfort when she has a headache, and she has never had a headache like this type before. She gets 8 hours of sleep a night, does not snore, and wakes up rested.

Exam: No cranial nerve deficits, including normal auditory in each ear, and the rest of the neurological exam is normal. Palpation of the right temple causes mild discomfort but does not illicit the same stabbing pain.
Additional diagnostic studies needed: MRI brain, ESR, CRP
Diagnosis: Cluster headache
Treatment: Oxygen

Case 1.2: Giant Cell Arteritis

A 85-year-old woman states that the headache started over the last month and is constant throughout the day. The headache occurs daily and feels like an ache all over her head but is noticeably worse on the right side of her head, and it is tender to the touch. She denies photophobia, phonophobia, and nausea. Chewing significantly worsens her headache and she feels pain in her right jaw. She has never had this type of headache before. She gets 8 hours of sleep a night, does not snore, and wakes up rested. She may have had a visual change in the right eye recently, which was described as "losing the top of her vision on the right."

Exam: No cranial nerve deficits and the rest of the neurological exam is normal. Applied pressure to each TMJ does not elicit pain. Pressure to the right temporalis yields severe pain.
Additional diagnostic studies needed: MRI brain, ESR, CRP, ophthalmology appointment with fluorescein angiography
Diagnosis: Giant cell arteritis
Treatment: High-dose steroids

1.5 Case Explanations

Case 1.1A demonstrates a patient with migraine without aura. There are some key aspects to this scenario that need clarification. The patient stated initially that this headache caused right ear pain and that she did not feel like eating. If the practitioner ignores the rest of the history and the physical exam, these facts meet many criteria for TMD. If this happens and the patient undergoes surgery for TMD, it is likely that the patient will continue to have headache after TMJ surgery. In this case, the ear pain is either referred pain from the unilateral onset of the headache; or it may be the patient's initial way of communicating that loud sounds worsen the headache. A mild pain response to palpation over the area of migraine is normal, which occurs in this case. Magnetic resonance imaging (MRI) of the brain as part of the workup would not be unreasonable given that the headache is new onset; however, the description is typical for migraine so the practitioner would not be faulted if an MRI is not obtained. In women, hormonal changes like menopause and postmenopause can cause migraine.

Case 1.1B demonstrates a patient with infrequent episodic TTH. If the practitioner fails to obtain an entire headache history, aspects of this case could lead to the misdiagnosis of TMD. Temporomandibular dysfunction pain is often a dull type of pain and causes ear pain and may be either unilateral or bilateral. The bilateral pain in TMD is the result of pain from the muscles of mastication. Tension-type headache can worsen when chewing foods with greater consistency. When foods that require minimal effort to chew induce pain, then the headache source may be the TMJ. In the case described, the patient clarifies that the pain does not originate from the ear, most foods do not worsen headache when chewing, and the practitioner has reassurance that the patient had this type of headache for many years.

Case 1.1C demonstrates a patient with trigeminal neuralgia. As previously mentioned, TMD pain is usually dull, and there is a dull component to the headache described in this case. In fact, the quality of the headache is not part of the diagnostic criteria for TMD. As a result, the patient in this case does meet the diagnostic criteria for TMD except for the last component mentioned in part D of Box 1.9, which states that the headache must not meet criteria for another diagnosis. Practitioners who treat patients for TMD or TMJ disorders must readily recognize trigeminal neuralgia in order to prevent the wrong diagnosis. Both forms of headache are closely related in presentation and triggers, and they involve the same structures and innervation. Specifically, pain sensation from the TMJ is innervated by the mandibular division of the trigeminal nerve [3, 4]. The primary difference between these two disorders is that patients with trigeminal neuralgia give a description of sharp, electric pain attacks that are brief. A residual dull ache is not unusual after a trigeminal neuralgia episode. MRI and MRA of the brain is reasonable in this case given the headache is of new onset and to evaluate if vasculature is irritating the trigeminal nerve, which may require a surgical treatment if pharmacotherapy does not work.

Box 1.9: Headache Attributed to Temporomandibular Disorder (TMD) [2]
Diagnostic criteria:

A. Any headache fulfilling criterion C
B. Clinical and/or imaging evidence of a pathological process affecting the temporomandibular joint (TMJ), muscles of mastication, and/or or associated structures
C. Evidence of causation demonstrated by at least two of the following:
   1. Headache has developed in temporal relation to the onset of the temporomandibular disorder
   2. Either or both of the following: (a) headache has significantly worsened in parallel with progression of the temporomandibular disorder and (b) headache has significantly improved or resolved in parallel with improvement in or resolution of the temporomandibular disorder
   3. The headache is produced or exacerbated by active jaw movements, passive movements through the range of motion of the jaw, and/or provocative maneuvers applied to temporomandibular structures such as pressure on the TMJ and surrounding muscles of mastication
   4. Headache, when unilateral, is ipsilateral to the side of the temporomandibular disorder
D. Not better accounted for by another ICHD-3 diagnosis

Case 1.1D demonstrates a patient with cluster headache. Magnetic resonance imaging of the brain is necessary given that the headache is of new onset. Erythrocyte sedimentation rate (ESR) and C-reactive protein (CRP) should also be ordered as the headache description could be giant cell arteritis, and if the practitioner fails to make the diagnosis of giant cell arteritis early, permanent blindness could result. If there is no response to oxygen therapy, then indomethacin should be tried given that hemicrania headaches may present in the same manner as cluster headaches. If there is full resolution of the headache and the headache does not return after initiation of indomethacin, the diagnosis is hemicrania headache for this case.

Case 1.2 demonstrates a patient with giant cell arteritis. The case in this scenario provides an interesting thought process about the various headache types discussed so far. This scenario could fit TTH that is now chronic, could fit trigeminal neuralgia, and could fit TMD. If inflammatory markers are elevated or suspicion remains high for giant cell arteritis with normal inflammatory markers, then there should be no delay in treatment and biopsy should be pursued. Therefore, the case in this scenario illustrates the importance of remaining vigilant for other causes of headache that appear to meet the criteria for TMD.

There are multiple reasons as to why a patient continues to have headache after TMJ surgery. These reasons include but are not limited to the wrong initial diagnosis, existence of more than one headache type, and depression. It is essential to consider other diagnoses and use a wide range of conservative treatments before surgical treatment.

Although TMJ surgery may reduce the frequency of migraine and TTH as TMD can trigger these headaches, TMJ surgery will not cure these headaches. Temporomandibular joint surgery is indicated to treat intra-articular sources of pain and limited range of motion. Surgery is beneficial when the correct diagnosis is made and appropriate surgery chosen. The persistence or development of myofascial pain, neuralgias, or other headaches as a result of the surgery should always be considered [16–18].

In clinical studies, postsurgery follow-up data suggests that anywhere from 13% to 25% of patients who have TMJ surgery still suffer from headache at least 1 year after surgery although the frequency is often lower [14, 16]. In another study, 40% of subjects had headache preoperatively with less than 5% having headache 2 years after surgery [15]. Patients with depression at baseline are more likely to have severe headache or TMD than patients without depression. A study of over 1000 patients found that severe headache or TMD maybe the first presentation of pain in a patient with depression [19]. The study found that patients with severe depression or chronic depression at baseline had a statistically significant higher rate of developing severe headache as a new onset pain syndrome. It also found that those patients with depression and an established pain syndrome had a statistically significant higher rate of developing severe headache or of developing TMD as another pain syndrome. This study reveals that there is an association between depression, headache, and TMD. If depression is left untreated, headache may continue even after TMJ surgery.

Summary

About half the US population has TMD but only 10% have a painful TMJ [3–5]. More than half of those individuals with a headache disorder meet the diagnostic criteria for TMD, with migraine and TTH having the highest prevalence in this population. TMD disorder involves the structures in the temporomandibular region, which are the TMJ and the muscles of mastication [5]. Due to this anatomical relationship, TMD may mimic multiple different types of headache including migraine, TTH, chronic daily headache, neoplasm, trigeminal neuralgia, giant cell arteritis, cluster headache, and cervicogenic headache. Recognizing these headache types and their differences will help prevent making the wrong diagnosis in a patient with a new onset headache. Some of the headaches that patients experience after TMJ surgery may be the result of initial misdiagnosis of TMD, patients having more than one headache type, or depression.

References

1. World Health Organization. Headache disorders. Fact sheet N 277. October 2012.
2. Headache Classification Committee of the International Headache Society (IHS). The International Classification of Headache Disorders, 3rd edition (beta version). Cephalalgia. 2013;33:629.
3. Graff-Radford S. Facial pain, cervical pain, and headache. Continuum. 2012;18:869.
4. Graff-Radford S, Bassiur J. Temporomandibular disorders and headaches. Neurologic Clin Second Headache. 2014;32:525.

5. LeResche L. Epidemiology of temporomandibular disorders: implications for the investigation of etiological factors. Crit Rev Oral Biol Med. 1997;8:291.
6. Ballegard V, Thede-Schmidt-Hansen P, Svensson P, et al. Are headache and temporomandibular disorders related? A blinded study. Cephalalgia. 2008;28:832.
7. Cooper B, Kleinberg I. Examination of a large patient population for the presence of symptoms and signs of temporomandibular disorders. Cranio. 2007;25:114.
8. Di Paolo C, Costanzo G, Panti F, et al. Epidemiological analysis on 2375 patients with TMJ disorders: basic statistical aspects. Ann Stomatol. 2013;4:161.
9. Scrivani S, Mehta N. Temporomandibular disorders in adults. Up-to-date 2016; Last accessed 2/29/16.
10. De Rossi S, Greenberg M, Liu F, et al. Temporomandibular disorders evaluation and management. Med Clin North Am. 2014;98:1353.
11. Bajwa Z, Ho C, Khan S. Trigeminal neuralgia. Up-to-date 2016; Last accessed 2/29/16.
12. Fromm G, Graff-Radford S, Terrence C, et al. Pre-trigeminal neuralgia. Neurology. 1990;40:1493.
13. Juniper R, Glynn C. Association between paroxysmal trigeminal neuralgia and atypical facial pain. Br J Oral Maxillofac Surg. 1999;37:444.
14. Mehra P, Wolford L. The Mitek mini anchor for TMJ disc repositioning: surgical technique and results. Int J Oral Maxillofac Surg. 2001;30:497.
15. Montgomery M, Gordon S, Van Sickels J, et al. Changes in signs and symptoms following temporomandibular joint disc repositioning surgery. J Oral Maxillofac Surg. 1992;50:320.
16. Panula K, Somppi M, Finne K, et al. Effects of orthognathic surgery on temporomandibular joint dysfunction. Int J Oral Maxillofac Surg. 2000;29:183.
17. Hoffman D, Puig L. Complications of TMJ surgery. Oral Maxillofac Surg Clin North Am. 2015;27:109.
18. Panula K, Finne K, Oikarinen K. Incidence of complications and problems telated to orthognathic surgery: a review of 655 patients. J Oral Maxillofac Surg. 2001;59:1128.
19. Von Korff M, Le Resche L, Dworkin S. First onset of common pain symptoms: a prospective study of depression as a risk factor. Pain. 1993;55:251.

Failure to Make the Correct Diagnosis: Part II – A Physical Therapist's Perspective

2

Steve Kraus

2.1 Introduction

The 2013 International Headache Society (IHS) has identified 14 diagnostic categories for headache and facial pain [1] (Appendix 1). Each of these categories have several diagnostic subtypes for a total of 284 sources for headache and facial pain. This extensive list of headache and facial pain disorders becomes a diagnostic challenge even for the most seasoned clinicians. A thorough history and a cranial nerve exam assessing neurological deficit(s) and/or altered mental state can eliminate more serious pathologies that may be causing headache and facial pain. If pathology or infection is suspected, imaging studies and blood analysis would rule out most concerns [2]. Neuropathic and neurogenic sources for headache and facial pain must be considered but are very complex and difficult to diagnose [3]. Category 11 of the IHS classification system addresses additional diagnoses that are relatively common and can mimic and compound temporomandibular joint pain (Boxes 2.1 and 2.2).

Electronic supplementary material The online version of this chapter (doi: 10.1007/978-3-319-51241-9_2) contains supplementary material, which is available to authorized users.

S. Kraus, PT
Division of Physical Therapy, Department of Rehabilitation Medicine, Emory University School of Medicine, Atlanta, GA, USA

The Georgia School of Orthodontics, Atlanta, GA, USA
e-mail: Steve.Kraus@myphysio.com

G.F. Bouloux (ed.), *Complications of Temporomandibular Joint Surgery*,
DOI 10.1007/978-3-319-51241-9_2

Box 2.1 Classification of Headache Disorders [1]

Part one: the primary headaches

1. Migraine
2. Tension type headache
3. Trigeminal autonomic cephalalgias
4. Other primary headache disorders

Part two: the secondary headaches

5. Headache attributed to trauma or injury to the head and/or neck
6. Headache attributed to cranial or cervical vascular disorder
7. Headache attributed to nonvascular intracranial disorder
8. Headache attributed to a substance or its withdrawal
9. Headache attributed to infection
10. Headache attributed to disorders of homeostasis
11. Headache or facial pain attributed to disorder of the cranium, neck, eyes, ears, nose, sinuses, teeth, mouth, or other facial or cervical structures
12. Headache attributed to psychiatric disorder

Part three: painful cranial neuropathies, other facial pains, and other headaches

13. Painful cranial neuropathies and other facial pains
14. Other headache disorders

Box 2.2 Diagnostic Subsets of Category 11 [1]

Headache or facial pain attributed to disorders of the cranium, neck, eyes, ears, nose, sinuses, teeth, mouth, or other facial or cervical structures

11.1	Headache attributed to disorder of cranial bone
11.2.1	*Cervicogenic headache*
11.2.2	Headache attributed to retropharyngeal tendonitis
11.2.3	Headache attributed to craniocervical dystonia
11.3	Headache attributed to disorder of the eyes
11.3.1	Headache attributed to acute glaucoma
11.3.2	Headache attributed to refractive error
11.3.3	Headache attributed to heterophoria or heterotropia
11.3.4	Headache attributed to ocular inflammatory disorder
11.3.5	Headache attributed to trochleitis
11.5	Headache attributed to disorder of the nose or paranasal sinuses
11.5.1	Headache attributed to acute rhinosinusitis
11.5.2	Headache attributed to chronic or recurrent rhinosinusitis
11.6	Headache attributed to disorder of the teeth or jaw
11.7	*Headache attributed to temporomandibular joint disorder (TMD)*
11.8	Headache attributed to inflammation of the stylohyoid ligament
11.9	Headache or facial pain attributed to other disorders of the cranium, neck, eyes, ears, nose, sinuses, teeth, mouth, or other facial or cervical structures

2.2 Diagnosing Headache and Facial Pain

One of the first manuscripts that purported to identify the cause of TMD was published by Coston in 1934 [4]. The loss of hearing, tinnitus, dizziness, headache, and a burning sensation of the throat and tongue were then thought to be the result of a dental malocclusion. The association between malocclusion and TMD remains very controversial for many reasons including the high prevalence of malocclusion in the general population [5]. At the present time, there is little evidence to support occlusion as a predisposing factor, nor is there any evidence to support occlusal equilibration, prosthodontics, and orthodontics in the prevention and treatment of TMD [6, 7]. Likewise occlusal interferences are not thought to result in the development of TMD and the treatment of interference is unlikely to result in resolution of TMD [6–11]. The etiology of TMD is clearly complex, and making the correct diagnosis in the face of so many potential sources of facial pain can be challenging [12].

2.3 Diagnostic Tests

An accurate diagnosis requires a reasonably reliable and reproducible diagnostic protocol that screens for multiple causes of facial pain. The history and physical examination remain critical to developing a differential diagnosis. Although advocated by some clinicians, the use of sonography, electromyography, myomonitoring, and kinesiology has little to offer for the diagnosis of TMD [13, 14]. Although the use of MRI of the TMJ to diagnose disc displacement or degenerative joint disease is reasonable, these pathological entities may not be responsible for pain and reduced function unless suggested by the history and clinical examination [15]. Disc displacements occur in nearly one third of asymptomatic and healthy subjects [16]. Imaging studies are necessary if the patient has failed to respond to conservative treatment for intra-articular disorders, and TMJ surgery is being considered.

The original Research Diagnostic Criteria for Temporomandibular Disorders (RDC/TMD) is the most widely used diagnostic protocol for researchers and clinicians to diagnose common diagnostic subsets of TMD [17]. The RDC/TMD diagnostic protocol is divided into Axis I that consists of the history and physical exam and Axis II which assesses related psychosocial dysfunction and psychological distress. In 2014, the RDC/TMD was renamed to the Diagnostic Criteria of Temporomandibular Disorders (DC/TMD) and was revised to present new evidence-based Axis I and Axis II diagnostic criteria for the 12 common TMDs [18]. Sensitivity and specificity values have been established for 10 of the 12 diagnostic subsets of TMD. Diagnostic protocols with a sensitivity of $\geq .70$ and specificity of $\geq .95$ are considered satisfactory. Currently only five of the ten subsets of TMD have diagnostic protocols with adequate sensitivity and specificity. The remaining five subsets of TMD do not have diagnostic protocols with satisfactory sensitivity and specificity values. The DC/TMD is intended for immediate implementation in clinical and research settings. Incorporating the DC/TMD criterion along with

Table 2.1 Diagnostic subset of TMD with sensitivity and specificity [14]

Myogenous	Sensitivity	Specificity
Myalgia	.90	.99
Local myalgia	N/A	N/A
Myofascial Pain	N/A	N/A
Myofascial pain with referral	.86	.98
Headache attributed to TMD	.89	.87
Arthrogenous		
Arthralgia	.89	.98
Disc displacement with reduction	.34	.92
Disc displacement with reduction and intermittent locking	.38	.98
Disc displacement without reduction with limited opening	.80	.97
Disc displacement without reduction without limited opening	.54	.79
Degenerative joint disease	.55	.61
Subluxation	.98	1.0

clinical reasoning and experience will guide the clinician to make an accurate diagnosis of TMD, including intra-articular pathology that may benefit from surgical intervention. (Table 2.1)

The diagnostic subsets of TMD are not mutually exclusive, and it is not uncommon to have patients with more than one diagnosis [19, 20]. The DC/TMD diagnostic criteria are based on the patient having singular Axis I diagnosis rather than multiple diagnostic subsets of TMD. Future versions of the DC/TMD will need to identify patients who meet criteria for multiple diagnostic subtypes. Failing to identify a patient with more than one subset of TMD may also result in treatment failure. It behooves clinicians to seek concurrent diagnostic subsets of TMD and other sources of facial pain in all patients.

2.4 Treatment

Reducing or eliminating pain is one of the cornerstones of having a successful treatment outcome for TMD [21]. The DC/TMD myogenous diagnostic subsets consisting of myalgia, local myalgia, myofascial pain, myofascial pain with referral, and headache attributed to TMD, although distinct, will be collectively be referred to as myalgia for the purpose of this discussion. Myalgia is the most prevalent diagnostic subset among all diagnostic subsets of TMD with arthralgia being the second most common diagnostic subset [21, 22]. The DC/TMD diagnostic criteria for myalgia and arthralgia requires pain to be present in the past 30 days. In addition pain must be present during the examination, and it must increase or decrease in response to provocation tests. This includes palpation to the muscles of mastication or TMJ capsule and/or pain that is modified by active or passive movements of the jaw.

The DC/TMD criterion for the remaining six intra-articular disorders (IADs) does not require pain to be present. These six IADs are diagnosed by patient complaints of noise or difficulty opening or closing their mouth. Though these symptoms can be annoying and disconcerting to the patient, they are often not painful [23]. An accurate diagnosis of the six IADs is necessary in order to educate the patient on their condition and provide a prognosis of their intra-articular disorder either with or without treatment. The diagnostic criteria for the remaining six IADs are as follows:

- *Disc displacement with reduction*
- In the past 30 days, patient has had joint noises (click) with jaw movement or function with noises present during the exam.
- *Disc displacement with reduction with intermittent locking*
- In the past 30 days, patient has had joint noises (click) with movement or function, and jaw has locked for a moment with limited mouth opening.
- *Disc displacement without reduction with limited mouth opening*
- Patient has a prior history of a disc displacement with reduction with or without intermittent locking. At the time of the exam, patient's jaw is locked, so the mouth cannot open all the way with limitations in jaw opening severe enough to limit jaw opening and interfere with the ability to eat.
- *Disc displacement without reduction without limited mouth opening*
- Patient has a prior history of a disc displacement without reduction with limited opening but currently no limitation in jaw opening.
- *Degenerative joint disease*
- At the time of the exam, joint noises (crepitus) with jaw movement.
- *Subluxation*
- In the past 30 days, patient complains of jaw locking or catching in a wide-open mouth position, even for a moment, so the patient could not close from the wide-open position and there is inability to close the mouth from a wide-open position without a self-maneuver.
- If pain is accompanying any of the six IADs, clinicians should first consider myalgia and/or arthralgia as the patient's primary source of pain. Myalgia and arthralgia should generally be viewed as mutually independent conditions unrelated to the six IADs [23, 24]. Achieving a satisfactory treatment outcome is initially dependent on making an accurate diagnosis of one or multiple TMD diagnostic subsets and differentiating between diagnostic subsets that are known to be painful (myalgia and arthralgia) from subsets that may or may not be painful (six IADs). Finally and equally important is developing a treatment plan that addresses the patients primary pain source.

2.5 Biopsychosocial Issues

Pain is a subjective experience that is dependent on peripheral and central modulation of the nociceptive input. Persistent nociceptive input leads to peripheral sensitization. Ongoing peripheral sensitization leads to central sensitization resulting in hyperalgesia or allodynia [25]. Central sensitization reflects the ability of the central nervous system to change, distort, inhibit, or amplify nociceptive input, a process referred to as neuroplasticity [26]. Neuroplasticity is dependent on how an individual processes nociceptive input. The central modulation of nociceptive input is further dependent on several factors including the patient's psychosocial makeup [27]. This has become known as the biopsychosocial model. As a result, an individual's genetic composition, prior learning history, current psychological state, and sociocultural factors all influence pain perception and experience. These same factors should be considered in treatment planning as two different patients with similar clinical examination findings and diagnoses may respond in very different ways to the same treatment.

Prior to the onset of pain, an individual can have varying degrees of fear, anxiety, anger, and/or depression. When pain develops, patients with TMD unfortunately often consult with many healthcare professionals. A patient may potentially not receive a diagnosis, or the patient may receive conflicting diagnoses that have conflicting treatment recommendations with variable costs. This may compound the patient's preexisting fear, anxiety, anger, and depression, or it can result in the development of these maladaptive behaviors [28] (Videos 2.1, 2.2, and 2.3). If the clinician recognizes that a patient has acquired an inaccurate belief of their condition or was exposed to misinformation from family, friends, coworkers, and unfortunately healthcare professionals, the clinician should be sensitive to the situation and address these inaccurate beliefs and misinformation. Inaccurate beliefs and enhanced emotions will affect the patient's response to provocation testing done during the exam and may result in incorrect diagnoses and ultimately inappropriate treatment. Axis II of the DC/TMD recommends several reliable questionnaires the patient can complete that will give the clinician insight into a patient's emotional state [29]. The importance of identifying Axis II diagnoses cannot be underestimated as these will have a significant impact on treatment outcomes unless recognized and managed appropriately.

2.6 Neck Pain

Disorders of the neck is recognized by the IHS (category 11, subtype category 11.2) as a source of headache and facial pain (Box 2.2). Cervical spine disorder (CSD) includes disc herniation, disc degeneration, central or peripheral nerve involvement, facet joint arthralgia, facet joint hypomobility, and myalgia. The prevalence of CSD is very common in the general population. Seventy percent of the population will have had neck pain at some point in their life; 54% will have had neck pain in the past 6 months, and the point prevalence of neck pain is estimated to be 16% [30]. It is not surprising that neck pain occurs concurrently in 70% of patients diagnosed with TMD [19, 31].

Although the cervical spine is recognized by the IHS as a source of headache, facial, jaw, and ear pain, it is often misdiagnosed or unrecognized (Videos 2.4 and 2.5). A headache originating from the cervical spine is referred to as a cervicogenic headache (CH) [32]. A CH is located at the base of the head/upper neck to extend to the forehead and retro-orbital area [33]. In severe cases, a CH can be associated with vomiting, nausea, and photophobia. These aforementioned symptoms are similar to migraine, cluster, benign paroxysmal hemicranias, hemicranias continua, and tension-type headaches.

Patients can have CH that is concurrent with other types of headache. Cervicogenic headache is most frequently seen with migraine. Overlap of symptoms between these two makes the differential diagnosis a challenge. Seventy percent of patients that have been diagnosed with migraine complain of neck pain [34]. Conversely, neck pain is a more common complaint than nausea for patients experiencing a migraine. Cervicogenic headache is also considered as a cause of migraine [35]. Furthermore the estimated prevalence of CH is 17.8% in a general population which is similar to that of migraine. [36]

The reason that CSD can be a source of headache and facial pain is based on the convergence of cervical and cranial sensory neurons. Nociceptive afferent input from cervical spine tissues innervated by C1, C2, and C3 and nociceptive afferent input from tissues innervated by the trigeminal nerve (CV), converge in the trigeminocervical nucleus (TN) [37]. The TN is the major nociceptive nucleus of the head, throat, and neck areas. This nucleus is continuous with the gray matter of the spinal dorsal horn at the C1, C2, and C3 levels [38]. This topographic arrangement of the TN allows for the greatest interchange of nociceptive input to occur with the ophthalmic division of the trigeminal nerve resulting in perceived pain in the areas of the forehead, temple, or orbit [33] (Videos 2.6, 2.7, and 2.8).

The diagnostic criteria for CSD and CH may require anesthetic blocks directed at the greater occipital nerve, lessor occipital nerve, and upper cervical facet joints when the clinical examination is equivocal or the response to conservative treatment is poor [39]. Imaging studies of the cervical spine are generally not necessary to diagnose CSD or CH. Asymptomatic subjects have positive magnetic resonance imaging (MRI) findings related to cervical spondylosis in 25% of subjects less than 40 years of age and 60% of subjects greater than 40 years of age [40]. The high prevalence of positive degenerative findings in asymptomatic individuals emphasizes that common degenerative findings on MRI cannot be assumed to be the primary cause of symptoms in adult patients with neck pain. Imaging studies are only necessary if the patient has not responded to evidence-based conservative care, and surgery is being considered.

A diagnostic criteria for CSD and CH is shown in Box 2.3. A detailed discussion of the physical exam for CSD and CH is beyond the scope of this paper, but a more detailed discussion of diagnosing CSD and CH can be found elsewhere [40–44]. The more common and overlooked source of CH that can be easily diagnosed is cervical myalgia (myofascial trigger points (MTrPs)) [45–53]. Active or latent MTrPs can only be diagnosed by palpation. Clinicians need to become familiar with cervical spine muscles including suboccipital, splenius capitis, sternocleidomastoid, and trapezius muscles and their pattern of pain referral to the head and face (Fig. 2.1). The objective of palpating MTrPs in the cervical spine muscles is to reproduce or increase the patient's neck, facial, jaw, or ear pain. Cervical spine disorder should also be suspected when the clinical examination does not support TMD; the patient has not responded to oral appliances, medication, and/or therapeutic injections; and common causes of facial pain have been eliminated.

Box 2.3 Diagnostic Criteria for Cervical Spine Disorders and Cervicogenic Headache

1. Neurological exam
   (a) Upper extremity reflex, cutaneous, and muscle strength testing
   (b) Upper limb tension test
   (c) Neck distraction test
   (d) Spurling's test
   (e) Hoffmann's reflex
2. Provocation, mobility, and strength tests
   (a) Passive intervertebral mobility testing of facet joints.
      (i) Increases patient's familiar pain
      (ii) Restricted or excessive mobility of a facet joint(s)
   (b) Palpation of the lateral margins of the facet joints C2 through C7 increases patient's familiar pain.
   (c) Cervical spine mobility of flexion, extension, side bending, and rotation.
      (i) Maximum active cardinal plane movements increase patient's familiar pain
      (ii) Restricted mobility in anyone or combination of cardinal plane movements
   (d) Weakness of the anterior cervical spine muscles.
   (e) Palpation of the cervical spine muscles for active or latent MTrPs increases patient's familiar pain.

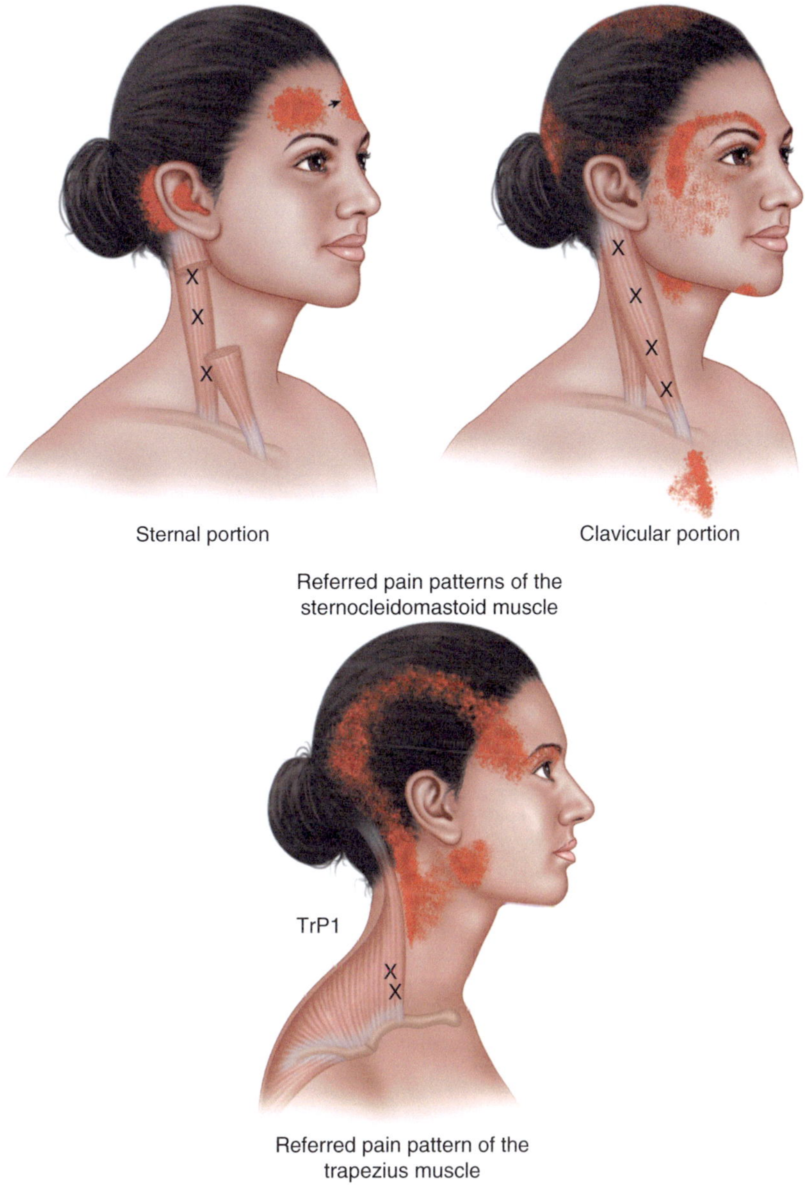

Fig. 2.1 Myofascial pain trigger points

Summary

Treatment outcomes can be affected if the diagnostic process does not differentiate among diagnostic subsets of TMD that require treatment from those that do not require treatment. Clinicians need to consider a patient's response to provocation tests can be affected by the patient's biopsychosocial makeup, thus skewing the diagnostic process and ultimately treatment outcome. Clinicians need to be aware of other conditions that can be mistakenly diagnosed as TMD. Neck pain is a common source of headache and facial pain that is often misdiagnosed by providers. Being aware of these categories can help clinicians make the correct diagnosis and therefore provide a higher quality of care for their patients.

References

1. Headache Classification Committee of the International Headache Society (IHS). The international classification of headache disorders, 3rd ed. Cephalalgia. 2013;33(9):629–808.
2. Chou R, Qaseem A, Owens DK, et al. Diagnostic imaging for low back pain: advice for high-value health care from the American College of Physicians. Ann Intern Med. 2011;154(3):181–9.
3. Marbach JJ. Is phantom tooth pain a deafferentation (neuropathic) syndrome? Part II: Psychosocial considerations. Oral Surg Oral Med Oral Pathol. 1993;75(2):225–32.
4. Costen JB. A syndrome of ear and sinus symptoms dependent upon disturbed function of the temporomandibular joint. Ann Otol Rhinol Laryngol. 1934;43:1–15.
5. Profitt WR, Epker BN, Ackerman JL. Systematic description of dentofacial deformities: the database. In: Bell WH, Profitt WR, White RP, editors. Surgical correction of dentofacial deformities, vol. 1. Philadelphia: WB Saunders; 1980. p. 105–54.
6. Gremillion HA. TMD and maladaptive occlusion: does a link exist? J Craniomandib Pract. 1995;13(4):205–6.
7. Cooper BC, International College of Cranio-Mandibular Orthopedics (ICCMO). Temporomandibular disorders: a position paper of the International College of Cranio-Mandibular Orthopedics (ICCMO). Cranio. 2011;29(3):237–44.
8. Koh H, Robinson PG. Occlusal adjustment for treating and preventing temporomandibular joint disorders. Cochrane Database Syst Rev. 2003;(1).
9. Gremillion H. The relationship between occlusion and TMD: an evidence-based discussion. J Evid Base Dent Pract. 2006;6:43–7.
10. Klasser GD, Greene CS. The changing field of temporomandibular disorders: what dentists need to know. J Can Dent Assoc. February 2009;75(1):49–53.
11. Xie Q, Li X, Xu X. The difficult relationship between occlusal interferences and temporomandibular disorder – insights from animal and human experimental studies. J Oral Rehabil. 2013;40:279–92.
12. Greene CS. The Etiology of Temporomandibular Disorders: Implication for Treatment. J Orofac Pain. 2001;15:93–105.
13. Mohl ND. Reliability and validity of diagnostic modalities for temporomandibular disorders. Adv Dent Res. August 1993;7:113–9.
14. Greene CS. The role of technology in TMD diagnosis. In: Laskin DM, Greene CS, Hylander WL, editors. TMDs – an evidence-based approach to diagnosis and treatment. Chicago: Quintessence Publishing Co; 2006. p. 193–202.
15. Petersson A. What you can and cannot see in TMJ imaging--an overview related to the RDC/TMD diagnostic system. J Oral Rehabil. 2010;37:771–8.

16. Aiken A, Bouloux G, Hudgins P. MR imaging of the temporomandibular joint. Magn Reson Imaging Clin N Am. 2012 Aug;20(3):397–412.
17. Dworkin SF, LeResche L. Research diagnostic criteria for temporomandibular disorders: review, criteria, examinations and specifications, critique. J Craniomandib Disord Facial Oral Pain. 1992;6:301–55.
18. Schiffman E, Ohrbach R, Truelove E, Look J, Anderson G, Goulet JP, et al. Diagnostic criteria for temporomandibular disorders (DC/TMD) for clinical and research applications: recommendations of the International RDC/TMD Consortium Network* and Orofacial Pain Special Interest Groupdagger. J Oral Facial Pain Headache. 2014;28:6–27.
19. Kraus S. Characteristics of 511 TMD patients referred for physical therapy. Oral Surg Oral Med Oral Pathol Oral Radiol. 2014;118:432–9.
20. Lobbezoo-Scholte AM, Lobbezzo F, Steenks MH, et al. Diagnostic subgroups of craniomandibular disorders, part II: symptom profiles. J Orofac Pain. 1995;9:37–43.. Latremoliere I, Woolf CJ. Central Sensitization: A Generator of Pain Hypersensitivity by Central Neural Plasticity. J Pain. 2009;10(9): 895–926.
21. Al-Hasson HK, Ismail AI, Ash Jr MM. Concerns of patients seeking treatment for TMJ dysfunction. J Prosthet Dent. 1986;56:217–21.
22. List T, Dworkin SF. Comparing TMD diagnoses and clinical findings at Swedish and US TMD centers using research diagnostic criteria for temporomandibular disorders. J Orofac Pain. 1996;10:240–53.
23. Naeije M, Te Veldhuis AH, Te Veldhuis EC, Visscher CM, Lobbezzo F. Disc displacement within the human temporomandibular joint: a systematic review of a 'noisy annoyance'. J Oral Rehabil. 2013;40:139–58.
24. Stegenga B. Osteoarthritis of the temporomandibular organ and its relationship with disc displacement. J Orofac Pain. 2001;15:193–205.
25. Dommerholt J, Shah J. Myofascial pain syndrome. In: Ballantyne JC, Rathmell JP, Fishman SM, editors. Bonica's management of pain. Baltimore: Lippincott, Williams & Williams; 2010. p. 450–71.
26. Petersen-Felix S, Curatolo M. Neuroplasticity – an important factor in acute and chronic pain. Swiss Med Wkly. 2002;132:273–8.
27. Gatchel RJ, Bo Peng Y, Peters ML, Fuchs PN. The biopsychosocial approach to chronic pain: scientific advances and future directions. Psychological Bulletin Am Psychol Assoc. 2007;Vol. 133(4):581–624.
28. Bonathan CJ, Zakrzewska JM, Love J, Williams AC. Beliefs and distress about orofacial pain: patient journey through a specialist pain consultation. J Oral Facial Pain Headache. 2014;28:223–32.
29. http://www.rdc-tmdinternational.org/TMDAssessmentDiagnosis/DCTMD.aspx.
30. Fejer R, Kyvik K, Hartvigsen J. The prevalence of neck pain in the world population: a systemic critical review of the literature. Eur Spine J. 2006;15(6):834–48.
31. Ciancaglini R, Testa M, Radaelli G. Association of neck pain with symptoms of TMD in the general adult population. Scand J Rehabil Med. 1999;31:17–22.
32. Sjaastad O, Fredriksen TA, Pfaffenrath V. Cervicogenic headache: diagnostic criteria. Headache. 1998;38:442–5.
33. Biondi DM. Cervicogenic headache: mechanisms, evaluation, and treatment strategies. JAOA. 2000;100(9 Suppl):S7–S14.
34. Calhoun AH, Ford S, Millen C, et al. The prevalence of neck pain in migraine. Headache. 2010;50:1273–7.
35. Shevel E, Spierings E. Cervical muscles in the pathogenesis of migraine headache. J Headache Pain. 2004;5(1):12–4.
36. Nilsson N. The prevalence of cervicogenic headache in a random population sample of 20-59 year olds. Spine. 1995;20(17):1884–8.
37. Piovesan EJ, Kowacs PA, Oshinsky MI. Convergence of cervical and trigeminal sensory afferents. Curr Pain Headache Rep. 2003;7:377–83.

38. Bogduk N. The neck and headaches. Neurol Clin. 2004 Feb;22(1):151–71.
39. Manchikanti L, et al. Evidence-based practice guidelines for interventional techniques in the management of chronic spinal pain. Pain Phys. 2003;6:3–81.
40. The Bone and joint fecade (2000–2010) task force on neck pain and its associated disorders. Spine. 2008;33:S4.
41. Jull G, Bogduk N, Marsland A. The accuracy of manual diagnosis for cervical zygapophysial joint pain syndromes. Med J Aust. 1988;148(5):233–6.
42. Viikari-Juntura E, et al. Validity of clinical tests in the diagnosis of root compression in cervical disc disease. Spine. 1989;14:253–7.
43. Tong, C. The Spurling's test and cervical radiculopathy. Spine. 2002;27(2):156–9
44. van Duijn J, van Duijn AJ, Nitsch W. Orthopedic manual physical therapy including thrust manipulation and exercise in the management of a patient with cervicogenic headache: a case report. J Man Manip Ther. 2007;15(1):10–24.
45. Mense S, Simons DG, Russell J. Muscle pain: understanding its nature, diagnosis, and treatment. N Engl J Med. 2001;344:1026–1027. March 29, 2001.
46. Fernández-de-Las-Peñas C, Galan-del-Rio F, Alonso-Blanco C, et al. Referred pain from muscle trigger points in the masticatory and neck-shoulder musculature in women with temporomandibular disorder. J Pain. 2010;11(12):1295–304.
47. Rocha CB, Sanchez TG. Efficacy of myofascial trigger point deactivation for tinnitus control. Braz J Otorhinolaryngol. 2012;78(6):21–6.
48. William S. Teachey. Otolaryngic myofascial pain syndromes. Curr Pain Headache Rep. 2004;8:457–62.
49. Calandre EP, Hidalgo J, Garcia-Leiva JM, Rico-Villademoros F. Trigger point evaluation in migraine patients: an indication of peripheral sensitization linked to migraine predisposition? Eur. J Neurol. 2006;13(3):244–9.
50. Hsieh YL, Kao MJ, Kuan TS, Chen SM, Chen JT, Hong CZ. Dry needling to a key myofascial trigger point may reduce the irritability of satellite MTrPs. Am J Phys Med Rehabil. 2007;86(5):397–403.
51. Fernández-de-Las-Peñas C, Cuadrado ML, Pareja JA. Myofascial trigger points, neck mobility and forward head posture in unilateral migraine. Cephalalgia. 2006;26:1061–70.
52. Fernández-de-Las-Peñas C, Alonso-Blanco C, Cuadrado ML, Pareja JA. Forward head posture and neck mobility in chronic tension-type headache: a blinded, controlled study. Cephalalgia. 2005;26:314–9.
53. Fernández-de-Las-Peñas C, Cuadrado ML, Pareja JA. Myofascial trigger points, neck mobility, and forward head posture in episodic tension-type headache. Headache. 2007;47:662–72.

Failure to Make the Correct Diagnosis: Part III – A Surgeon's Perspective

3

Pushkar Mehra, Mohammed Nadershah, and Gary F. Bouloux

3.1 Introduction

The complex anatomy and function of the temporomandibular joint (TMJ) and its close proximity to adjacent tissues may explain the wide spectrum of disorders involving this joint. It is often hard to identify the exact cause of TMJ pain or the factors that perpetuate the pain and dysfunction. In general, it is important to differentiate whether the symptomatology is the result of an extra-articular or intra-articular process as this can often aid in developing an appropriate differential diagnosis and treatment plan.

3.2 Making the Correct Diagnosis

A detailed pain history from the patient that addresses the onset, severity, progression, quality, radiation, and presence or absence of any aggravating and alleviating factors is crucial. A history of spontaneous or iatrogenic occlusal changes including orthodontics, orthognathic surgery, and dental prosthodontic work should be also noted. Signs

P. Mehra, BDS, DMD, FACS (✉)
Department of Oral and Maxillofacial Surgery, Boston University, Henry M. Goldman School of Dental Medicine, Boston, MA, USA

Oral and Maxillofacial Surgery, Boston Medical Center and Beth Israel Deaconess Medical Center, Boston, MA, USA
e-mail: pmehra@bu.edu

M. Nadershah, BDS, MD
Oral and Maxillofacial Surgery, King Abdul Aziz University, Jeddah, Saudi Arabia

G.F. Bouloux, MD, DDS, MDSc, FRACDS(OMS), FACS
Division of Oral and Maxillofacial Surgery, Department of Surgery, Emory University School of Medicine, Atlanta, GA, USA
e-mail: gfboulo@emory.edu

G.F. Bouloux (ed.), *Complications of Temporomandibular Joint Surgery*,
DOI 10.1007/978-3-319-51241-9_3

such as joint noises, locking, and decrease in mandibular range of motion may all suggest an intra-articular disorder. Temporomandibular joint pain may be the result of internal derangement, inflammation of the synovial lining, other pathologies, or a combination of these. Involvement of multiple joints should alert the surgeon to the possibility of a systemic arthritide or condition. Altered sensation, unplanned weight loss, and hearing disturbances may be associated with a malignant TMJ process.

The clinical evaluation of the head and neck should include an examination of the muscles and TMJs and assessment for any asymmetry or skeletal deformity. An asymmetry of the facial skeleton, especially the mandible, might suggest a progressive overgrowth or resorption of one or both TMJs. Mandibular maximum interincisal opening (MIO) and excursive movements (lateral and protrusive) should accompany a thorough intraoral examination of the occlusion. Positive findings of parafunction such as signs of excessive occlusal wear facets and tongue crenations should be documented.

It is imperative that an accurate diagnosis be made prior to contemplating any nonsurgical or surgical treatment for TMJ disorders. The history and clinical examination remain the most important sources of information on which to make the correct diagnosis. Radiological imaging techniques may also be of additional help in making a correct diagnosis. In contrast to conventional imaging techniques that only provide structural information, advanced techniques like magnetic resonance scanning (MRI) and computerized tomography (CT) represent the gold standard in contemporary TMJ imaging for soft- and hard-tissue abnormalities, respectively. Additionally, nuclear imaging using radioactive isotopes offers a physiologic evaluation of the TMJ including information about active processes like inflammation, growth, or malignancy. These techniques may also allow for early detection of the condition prior to structural changes [1, 2]. Examples of this technology include single-photon emission computed tomography with technetium 99 methylene diphosphonate (SPECT/Tc-99 MDP), which gives three-dimensional images due to multiplanar imaging acquisition, and positron emission tomography (PET), which utilizes F-2-fluoro-2-deoxy-glucose, and can also be combined with CT images (PET/CT) for better anatomical correlation [3].

3.3 The Diagnostic Challenge

Identifying the correct diagnosis allows the surgeon to anticipate the natural progression of the disease as well as provide treatment directed by evidence-based guidelines. Some of the more challenging diagnostic dilemmas include the following:

- Arthralgia as a result of the inflammatory milieu versus the disc position
- Condylar enlargement conditions
- Condylar resorptive processes
- Clinical conditions mimicking TMJ closed lock
- Open lock

3.3.1 Arthralgia

Our understanding of temporomandibular joint arthralgia has increased significantly over the last 40 years. The contribution of inflammatory cytokines to the development of arthralgia has become apparent as a result of synovial sampling. Multiple cytokines including IL-1 beta, IL-8, IL-17, CXCL-1, CCL-20, TNF-α, IFN-γ, and TIMP-1 have been identified and found to correlate with pain, response to treatment, and/or the presence of internal derangement [4, 5]. Other interleukins also present possess anti-inflammatory properties including IL-4, IL-6, IL-10, IL-12, IL-13, and OCIF/OPG [6]. The net result of the inflammatory process is the generation of reactive oxygen species including myeloperoxidase, superoxide ion, hydrogen peroxide, hydroxyl radical, and peroxynitrite anion. The result is the development of chondromalacia and degenerative joint disease. The inflammatory process also results in the release of VEGF, NGF, and FGF leading to changes in the synovial vascularity usually presenting as hyperemia and synovitis. The possibility that chronic inflammation results in a reduction of the biomechanical properties of the fibrocartilage, disc, and bone leading to disc displacement and/or degenerative changes cannot be excluded [7]. However, the potential for disc displacement in an otherwise susceptible individual to lead to inflammation and/or degeneration cannot be excluded.

The presence of inflammation within the TMJ also appears to correlate with the presence of inflammatory biomarkers in the serum and saliva [8, 9]. The presence of inflammatory mediators within the temporomandibular joint and the correlation with pain provides an opportunity to treat these patients with anti-inflammatory medications. When patients fail to respond to systemic medication or when patients present with arthralgia and closed lock, the utility of arthrocentesis and arthroscopy becomes apparent. With few exceptions these procedures should be considered in most patients prior to any open procedure.

Although TMJ arthralgia can be explained by the presence of inflammatory mediators within the joint and/or disc position and health, the potential for peripheral and central sensitization to develop should not be underestimated [10, 11]. The presence of certain genetic polymorphisms may also predispose individuals to TMD. Furthermore multiple physiological and psychological domains may contribute to the development of TMD as well as multisystem dysregulation which is often seen in the same population [12, 13].

It seems prudent to proceed cautiously with any patient with temporomandibular joint arthralgia or closed lock first assuming that the pain is secondary to inflammation. Treatment strategies such as arthrocentesis and arthroscopy should be considered first. Arthroplasty to address disc position or structural abnormalities should be considered when the previous modalities have failed. Taking time to know the patient and carefully evaluating the response to prior surgical intervention will also allow the surgeon to develop rapport and identify comorbid psychological and physiological conditions that may make the patient a poor surgical candidate.

3.3.2 Enlarged Condyle

History

A 27-year-old adult patient was treated by an experienced surgeon with standard two-jaw orthognathic surgery. The initial preoperative clinical examination revealed an open bite on the left side. Postsurgically the occlusion was noted to be as planned, but a left-sided open bite was again noted at 24 months (Fig. 3.1a).

Diagnostic Error

The patient had a progressive facial asymmetry due to an active osteochondroma of the left TMJ, which was not diagnosed. The left condyle was significantly larger than the right side (Fig. 3.1b–d). This should have been investigated further with serial clinical examinations and an advanced imaging technique prior to jaw surgery.

Differential Diagnosis

The differential diagnosis of a unilateral enlarged condyle includes condylar hyperplasia (CH), hemimandibular hypertrophy (HH), hemimandibular elongation (HE), and osteochondroma. The clinical presentation may include a malocclusion with unilateral posterior open bite on the affected side, shifted dental midline and chin to contralateral side, canting of the occlusal plane, and progressive facial asymmetry

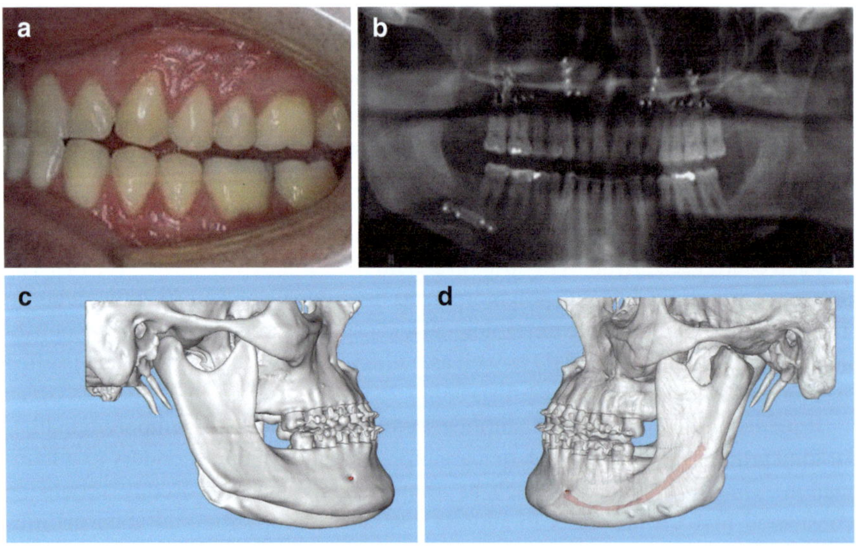

Fig. 3.1 (**a**) Intraoral photograph of a patient showing redevelopment of a left-sided open bite approximately 12 months after two-jaw orthognathic surgery. (**b**) Panoramic radiograph of the same patient after the orthognathic procedure (Note: The plate in the left mandible was removed due to a postoperative infection.) (**c**) 3-D reconstruction of right TMJ. The condyle appears normal in morphology. (**d**) 3-D reconstruction of left TMJ. Note the significantly larger and lobulated condyle, which is abnormal in shape

secondary to vertical elongation of the face on the affected side. Compensatory maxillary changes can accompany the displacement of the mandibular position in long-standing cases. Although CT scans and MRI examination may be used to supplement the work-up of such condylar pathology, it may be challenging to identify the diagnosis on the basis of clinical and radiographic assessment alone. An exophytic mass and a condylar head that is lobulated suggest osteochondroma, while an enlarged and elongated condyle may suggest CH, HH, or HE. A definitive diagnosis can only be made when the clinical and radiographic features are correlated with the histopathology.

Management Considerations

The first step in the treatment is to decide whether the enlarged condyle is still active and growing. If inactive, the patient can be treated with traditional orthognathic surgery with a realistic expectation of stability. If still active based on clinical, radiographic, or scintigraphic/PET scanning, it becomes important to make the correct diagnosis in order to determine the most appropriate surgical treatment. *High condylectomy* is a procedure in which 3–5 mm of the superior aspect of the condylar head is removed in an attempt to remove the cartilaginous cap. This is potentially a reasonable treatment choice to arrest active condylar hyperplasia but would not be appropriate for osteochondroma. *Low condylectomy* may be the treatment of choice in situations where the lesion involves the superior region of the condyle [14]. It has the advantage of preserving a portion of the joint while avoiding the need for joint reconstruction. However, there is little long-term data to support this approach. Resection of the condyle or osteochondroma involves a *complete condylectomy*, and while this eliminates all growth-related pathology, it does require either autogenous or alloplastic reconstruction [15].

3.3.3 Small Condyle

History

A 22-year-old patient was referred by her dentist to an orthodontist for evaluation and management of a worsening class II, open bite deformity which was also associated with TMJ pain and dietary limitations. She underwent a combined orthodontic and two-jaw surgical treatment with good results (Fig. 3.2a, b). Several months after debanding, she started to develop an anterior open bite again. Ultimately, there was significant degenerative change within bilateral TMJs (Fig. 3.2c) due to continued condylar resorption resulting in progressive mandibular retrusion (Fig. 3.2d, e).

Diagnostic Error

The patient had pre-existing, active TMJ condylar degeneration which was a source of the developing open bite and a progressive class II dentofacial deformity. In the presence of an active resorptive disease process, relapse and redevelopment of the malocclusion should have been expected.

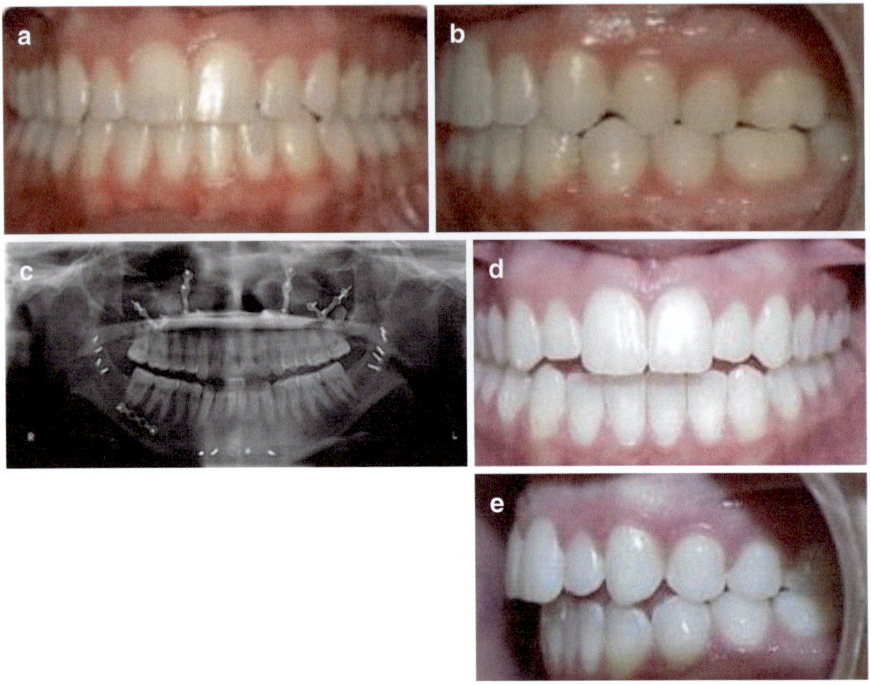

Fig. 3.2 (**a**, **b**) Intraoral views of the 8-month postoperative occlusion of a patient (immediately after removal of orthodontic appliances) who underwent combined orthodontic and orthognathic surgical treatment for correction of an open bite, class II skeletal and occlusal deformity. (**c**) Sixteen-month postoperative panoramic radiograph showing advanced bilateral resorption of condyles. (**d**, **e**) Relapse has occurred 4 months later due to continued TMJ condylar resorption

Differential Diagnosis

Evidence of condylar resorption in a young person manifested by a progressive change in occlusion or radiographic evidence of TMJ degeneration should alert the surgeon to the potential for progressive condylar resorption (PCR) or a systemic arthritide unless proven otherwise. Specific causes of condylar degeneration include rheumatoid arthritis, internal derangement, use of steroids, trauma, systemic autoimmune/connective tissue (CT) diseases (e.g., lupus, psoriasis, scleroderma), orthodontic treatment, and orthognathic surgery [16, 17].

Management Considerations

The etiology and pathogenesis of condylar resorption remains unclear. It may be classified into primary (idiopathic) and secondary (known etiology) depending on the presence of predisposing factors [18]. In PCR, the patient usually presents with a progressively retruded chin, mild TMJ pain with and open bite deformity. In contrast, many patients with TMJ resorption due to CT disease have significant preauricular joint and myofascial pain. Connective tissue diseases that can affect the TMJ are broadly divided into rheumatoid arthritis (RA) and the seronegative spondyloarthropathies. The latter can include conditions such as psoriatic arthritis, lupus arthritis, scleroderma, ankylosing spondylitis, arthritis associated with inflammatory bowel disease, and reactive arthritis. Juvenile idiopathic arthritis can be positive or negative for rheumatoid factor and also affects the TMJ in younger individuals leading to destruction of the condylar growth center with subsequent disturbances in mandibular growth [19, 20]. The metabolic diseases of gout and pseudo gout are also similarly known to affect the TMJ. The effects of these systemic autoimmune/CT diseases on the TMJ may induce a plethora of characteristic radiographic (MRI) findings such as abnormal disc position, abnormal disc morphology, osseous changes in the mandibular condyle, deformity of the articular eminence, and glenoid fossa, besides an abnormal bone marrow signal of the mandibular condyle [21]. If a patient is suspected to be having TMJ disorder secondary to a CT disease, rheumatology consultation is recommended.

If the resorption occurs in a bilateral fashion, there is a symmetric posterior shift of the mandible with class II skeletal and dental malocclusion. On the other hand, asymmetric bilateral or unilateral disease processes may result in a dental and skeletal mandibular midline shift, contralateral posterior open bite, and ipsilateral cross bite. Irrespective of the etiology, it is critical to determine whether the disease is active or not by a thorough history and serial clinical and radiographic evaluations. Computed scans and MRI provide static information and cannot provide information about disease activity. A technetium 99 MDP study can be useful in determining metabolic activity in the condyles. The treatment of TMJ condylar resorption remains controversial and will depend on the extent and stage of the disease. Although it may occasionally be self-limiting, it can be reactivated by orthodontics or orthognathic surgery [22–24]. Most clinicians agree that the TMJs must be stable prior to any orthognathic surgery. Potential treatments for patients with active PCR patients include the following: (1) *observation for disease arrest ("burn out")* followed by maxillary orthognathic surgery to close the open bite and/or chin camouflage surgery to improve facial profile, (2) *TMJ replacement with autogenous tissues* (most commonly costochondral grafts) with delayed orthognathic surgery, and (3) *TMJ replacement with alloplastic joints* with delayed or concomitant orthognathic surgery.

3.3.4 Clinical Conditions Mimicking TMJ Closed Lock

History

A 48-year-old adult patient had a history of progressively decreasing mouth opening over a period of 10 years with no TMJ pain and mild unilateral, left-sided temporal and masseter tenderness. When he presented initially to a local surgeon, he had a maximal inter-incisal opening of 16 mm. A preoperative panorex was unremarkable, and the surgeon prescribed NSAIDS and muscle relaxants and referred him for physical therapy without much success. A TMJ MRI was next obtained which showed bilateral internal derangement. The patient underwent bilateral TMJ arthrocentesis with no improvement.

Diagnostic Error

The etiology of the limited opening in this patient was a unilateral osteochondroma of the coronoid process, which was not diagnosed. The lack of joint pain and long-standing history should have alerted the clinician to other causes of limited opening. A CT scan may have been more beneficial than a MRI (Fig. 3.3a, b).

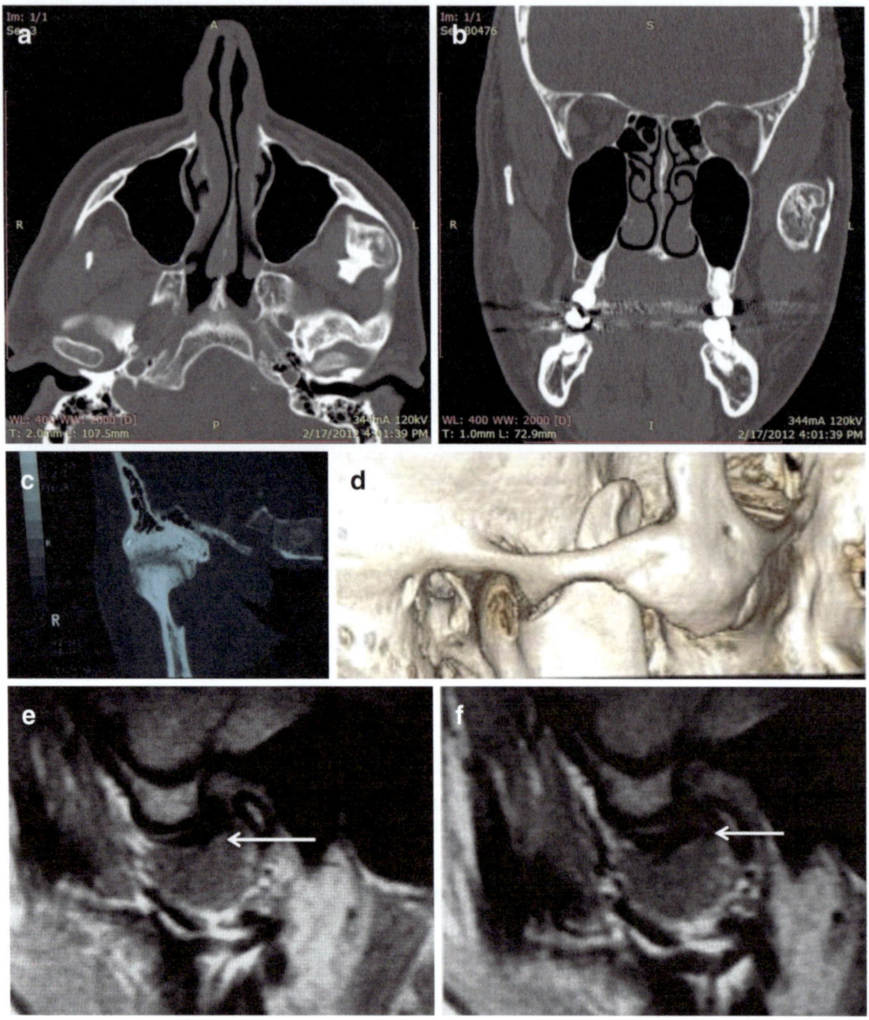

Fig. 3.3 (**a**) Axial CT scan showing an osteochondroma of the left mandibular coronoid process. (**b**) Coronal CT scan showing osteochondroma of the coronoid area which was causing impingement on the zygomatic arch during mandibular translation. (**c**, **d**) Other osseous etiologies of refractory trismus include TMJ ankylosis (c) and coronoid hyperplasia (d). (**e**) MRI image demonstrating closed mouth position with anteriorly displaced disc (*white arrow*). (**f**) Open mouth view of same patient showing limited mandibular translation and no mobility of displaced disc, which remains in the same position (beneath the articular eminence) as in the previous figure (*white arrow*)

Differential Diagnosis

Intra-articular TMJ disorders such as internal derangement, fibrous adhesions, and fibrous or bony ankylosis should be considered (Fig. 3.3c). Extra-articular conditions like coronoid hyperplasia (Fig. 3.3d) and neuromuscular disorders should also be considered.

Management Considerations

Prior to attempting any surgical treatment, it should be determined whether the hypomobility is intra-articular or extra-articular. The latter is a result of fibrosis and scarring of the muscles and soft tissues or mechanical impingement that is independent of the TMJ. This includes prior soft tissue trauma or surgery, radiation therapy [25, 26], depressed zygomatic arch fracture [27], myositis ossificans traumatica [28], severe facial burns, and coronoid hyperplasia [29]. The treatment of these conditions includes correction of the causative factor if possible and early aggressive physical therapy to improve the mandibular range of motion.

An acute intra-articular cause of limited opening may include closed lock secondary to internal derangement. Patients often present with limited inter-incisal opening and deviation to the affected side. Clicks are rarely encountered on exam, but patients may give a past history of them since there is often anterior disc displacement without reduction at the time of presentation (Fig. 3.3e, f). Pain is elicited when attempting to increase the opening by stretching or forcing. Treatment may include arthrocentesis or arthroscopy. An anchored disc may also cause limited opening despite normal disc position.

Long-term limited opening should alert the surgeon to multiple potential causes. The treatment of bony ankylosis varies according to the degree of ankylosis, surgeon experience, and preference. A variety of surgical techniques have been described in the literature with no single method proven to be ideal. This includes gap arthroplasty, interpositional arthroplasty, and TMJ reconstruction using autogenous or alloplastic replacements. Fibrous ankylosis may be amenable to be more conservative surgical management [30].

3.3.5 Increased or Normal Mouth Opening with Locked Jaw

History

An 18-year-old patient presented to the emergency room with a TMJ open lock condition. He gave a history of recurrent open locks during range of motion movements multiple times during the last 3 months, all of which were self-reducible. A CT scan was obtained and the patient was diagnosed as having a TMJ dislocation. The "dislocated mandible was reduced" under intravenous sedation by the ER physician. He was then referred to a specialist for follow-up.

Diagnostic Error

The clinician failed to diagnose the condition appropriately. The history of recurrent yet "self-reducible" open locks should have alerted the physician that the etiology was unlikely to be dislocated condyle out of the fossa and trapped anterior to the

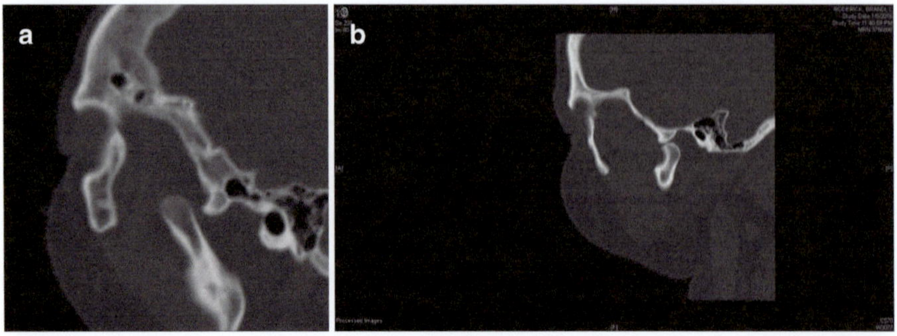

Fig. 3.4 (**a**) CT scan demonstrating true condylar dislocation with the mandibular condyle displaced beyond the anatomic limits of the glenoid fossa and is trapped anterior to the articular eminence. (**b**) CT scan showing that the mandibular condyle remains within the anatomic limits of the glenoid fossa and is not trapped anterior to the articular eminence

eminence. The CT scan obtained at the time of the locking (Fig. 3.4b) reveals that the condyle was not dislocated out of the fossa.

Differential Diagnosis

Open lock may be the result of either dislocation of the condyle (Fig. 3.4a) or a disc-condyle issue. In the former, there is usually hypermobility with steep articular eminence where the condyle gets trapped anterior to the fossa on wide opening, while in the latter, the condyle stays in the fossa (Fig. 3.4b) but translates anterior to the disc, which prevents closure.

Management Considerations

In TMJ condylar dislocation, the condyle is anterior and superior to the articular eminence on CT scan, and this condition is often accompanied by spasm of the muscles of mastication. Dislocation can be classified into acute or chronic, partial or complete, dislocation. Acute cases are typically managed by manual reduction and analgesics. On the other hand, chronic dislocation is managed by different nonsurgical and surgical options. Surgical treatment generally aims at either augmenting (to prevent dislocation) or removing the mechanical obstacle (to allow self-reduction).

In contrast to this scenario, there are some patients where the open lock condition occurs within the expected range of condylar motion [31]. In these cases, the occurrence of open lock is often spontaneous, and usually there is no associated history of joint laxity, neurologic disorders, and other factors that predispose to condylar dislocation [22]. On radiographic examination, the eminence is shallow and the condyle is located inferior to rather than in front of and superior to the eminence (Fig. 3.4b). The obstruction, which is not visible in plain radiographs or CT scans, may be demonstrated on TMJ MRI scans (esp. dynamic cine MRI) which show that the condyle is located in front of the anterior band of the disc in an open lock position and is unable to return posteriorly into the fossa due to mechanical obstruction by the disc. These cases can usually successfully be managed by arthrocentesis or disc-related surgical procedures.

References

1. Roh HS, Kim W, Kim YK, Lee JY. Relationships between disk displacement, joint effusion, and degenerative changes of the TMJ in TMD patients based on MRI findings. J Craniomaxillofac Surg. 2012;40:283–6.
2. Becker W, Meller J. The role of nuclear medicine in infection and inflammation. Lancet Infect Dis. 2001;1:326–33.
3. Coutinho A, Fenyo-Pereira M, Dib LL, Lima EN. The role of SPECT/CT with 99mTc-MDP image fusion to diagnose temporomandibular dysfunction. Oral Surg Oral Med Oral Pathol Oral Radiol Endod. 2006;101:224–30.
4. Bouloux GF. Temporomandibular joint pain and synovial fluid analysis: a review of the literature. J Oral Maxillofac Surg. 2009;67:2497–504.
5. Hattori T, Ogura N, Akutsu M, et al. Gene expression profiling of IL-17A-treated synovial fibroblasts from the human temporomandibular joint. Mediators Inflamm. 2015;2015: 436067.
6. Kellesarian SV, Al-Kheraif AA, Vohra F, et al. Cytokine profile in the synovial fluid of patients with temporomandibular joint disorders: a systematic review. Cytokine. 2016;77:98–106.
7. Wang XD, Cui SJ, Liu Y, et al. Deterioration of mechanical properties of discs in chronically inflamed TMJ. J Dent Res. 2014;93:1170–6.
8. Cevidanes LH, Walker D, Schilling J, et al. 3D osteoarthritic changes in TMJ condylar morphology correlates with specific systemic and local biomarkers of disease. Osteoarthritis Cartilage. 2014;22:1657–67.
9. Park JW, Chung JW. Inflammatory cytokines and sleep disturbance in patients with temporomandibular disorders. J Oral Facial Pain Headache. 2016;30:27–33.
10. Cady RJ, Glenn JR, Smith KM, Durham PL. Calcitonin gene-related peptide promotes cellular changes in trigeminal neurons and glia implicated in peripheral and central sensitization. Mol Pain. 2011;7:94.
11. Woolf CJ. Central sensitization: implications for the diagnosis and treatment of pain. Pain. 2011;152:S2–15.
12. Smith SB, Mir E, Bair E, et al. Genetic variants associated with development of TMD and its intermediate phenotypes: the genetic architecture of TMD in the OPPERA prospective cohort study. J Pain. 2013;14:T91–101.e1–3.
13. Chen H, Nackley A, Miller V, Diatchenko L, Maixner W. Multisystem dysregulation in painful temporomandibular disorders. J Pain. 2013;14:983–96.
14. Wolford LM, Movahed R, Dhameja A, Allen WR. Low condylectomy and orthognathic surgery to treat mandibular condylar osteochondroma: a retrospective review of 37 cases. J Oral Maxillofac Surg. 2014;72:1704–28.
15. Mehra P, Arya V, Henry C. Temporomandibular Joint Condylar Osteochondroma: complete condylectomy and joint replacement versus low condylectomy and joint preservation. J Oral Maxillofac Surg. 2016;74:911–25.
16. Kerstens HC, Tuinzing DB, Golding RP, van der Kwast WA. Condylar atrophy and osteoarthrosis after bimaxillary surgery. Oral Surg Oral Med Oral Pathol. 1990;69:274–80.
17. Papadaki ME, Tayebaty F, Kaban LB, Troulis MJ. Condylar resorption. Oral Maxillofac Surg Clin North Am. 2007;19:223–34, vii.
18. de Bont LG, Stegenga B. Pathology of temporomandibular joint internal derangement and osteoarthrosis. Int J Oral Maxillofac Surg. 1993;22:71–4.
19. Scolozzi P, Bosson G, Jaques B. Severe isolated temporomandibular joint involvement in juvenile idiopathic arthritis. J Oral Maxillofac Surg. 2005;63:1368–71.
20. Muller L, Kellenberger CJ, Cannizzaro E, et al. Early diagnosis of temporomandibular joint involvement in juvenile idiopathic arthritis: a pilot study comparing clinical examination and ultrasound to magnetic resonance imaging. Rheumatology (Oxford). 2009;48:680–5.
21. Abramowicz S, Cheon JE, Kim S, Bacic J, Lee EY. Magnetic resonance imaging of temporomandibular joints in children with arthritis. J Oral Maxillofac Surg. 2011;69:2321–8.

22. Hoppenreijs TJ, Freihofer HP, Stoelinga PJ, Tuinzing DB, van't Hof MA. Condylar remodelling and resorption after Le Fort I and bimaxillary osteotomies in patients with anterior open bite. A clinical and radiological study. Int J Oral Maxillofac Surg. 1998;27:81–91.
23. Arnett GW, Milam SB, Gottesman L. Progressive mandibular retrusion – idiopathic condylar resorption. Part I. Am J Orthod Dentofacial Orthop. 1996;110:8–15.
24. Arnett GW, Milam SB, Gottesman L. Progressive mandibular retrusion-idiopathic condylar resorption. Part II. Am J Orthod Dentofacial Orthop. 1996;110:117–27.
25. Dijkstra PU, Huisman PM, Roodenburg JL. Criteria for trismus in head and neck oncology. Int J Oral Maxillofac Surg. 2006;35:337–42.
26. Dijkstra PU, Kalk WW, Roodenburg JL. Trismus in head and neck oncology: a systematic review. Oral Oncol. 2004;40:879–89.
27. Rikalainen R, Lamberg MA, Tasanen A. Extra-articular fibrous ankylosis of the mandible after zygomatic fracture. J Maxillofac Surg. 1981;9:132–6.
28. Aoki T, Naito H, Ota Y, Shiiki K. Myositis ossificans traumatica of the masticatory muscles: review of the literature and report of a case. J Oral Maxillofac Surg. 2002;60:1083–8.
29. Tieghi R, Galie M, Piersanti L, Clauser L. Bilateral hyperplasia of the coronoid processes: clinical report. J Craniofac Surg. 2005;16:723–6.
30. Long X, Li X, Cheng Y, et al. Preservation of disc for treatment of traumatic temporomandibular joint ankylosis. J Oral Maxillofac Surg. 2005;63:897–902.
31. Nitzan DW. Temporomandibular joint "open lock" versus condylar dislocation: signs and symptoms, imaging, treatment, and pathogenesis. J Oral Maxillofac Surg. 2002;60:506–11; discussion 12–3.

Perforation of the External Auditory Canal or Middle Cranial Fossa

4

Gary Warburton and Nawaf Aslam-Pervez

4.1 Introduction

Open and arthroscopic surgeries of the temporomandibular joint (TMJ) are common and effective treatments for selected patients with TMJ disorders. However, complications inevitably occur, even in the hands of experienced TMJ surgeons. An understanding of the surrounding anatomy, as well as a knowledge of the potential complications, is essential and not only helps in avoiding these complications but also in their recognition and appropriate management, when they do occur. The TMJ is located in a complex anatomical region within the head and neck. It is bounded posteriorly by the external auditory canal and superiorly by the middle cranial fossa. Consequently these structures are at risk during open surgery and arthroscopy with the potential for serious complications.

4.2 Perforation of the External Auditory Canal (EAC)

4.2.1 Pathophysiology

The external auditory canal (EAC) runs from the auricle to the tympanic membrane. The EAC does not follow a straight course, but rather an S shape, first curving posterosuperiorly then anteroinferiorly. The EAC is angled toward the TMJ and lies in very close proximity as can be seen on computed tomography (CT) (Fig. 4.1).

The EAC is divided into two parts. The outer third has cartilaginous walls and the inner two-thirds have bony walls. The cartilaginous EAC is continuous with the auricular cartilage and has a fibrous attachment to the rim of the bony meatus.

G. Warburton, DDS, MD, FDSRCS, FACS (✉)
N. Aslam-Pervez, MB ChB, BA, B. Dent. Sc, MRCSI
Oral & Maxillofacial Surgery, University of Maryland Dental School, Baltimore, MD, USA
e-mail: gwarburton@umaryland.edu

G.F. Bouloux (ed.), *Complications of Temporomandibular Joint Surgery*,
DOI 10.1007/978-3-319-51241-9_4

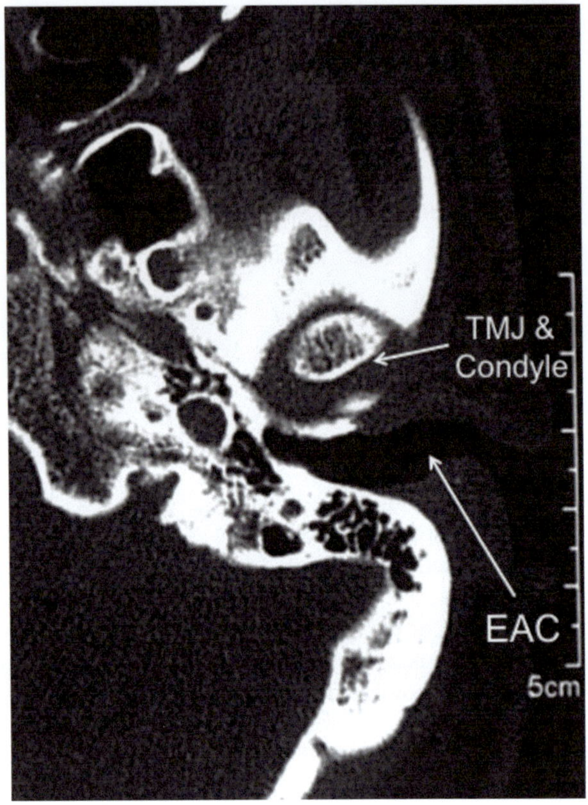

Fig. 4.1 Axial CT showing course of the EAC and TMJ proximity

The bony canal is mostly composed of the C-shaped tympanic portion of the temporal bone, and the superior wall is the squamous and petrous parts of the temporal bone. Foramen tympanicum (foramen of Huschke) in the tympanic plate of the temporal bone normally closes by 5 years of age, but may persist in up to 18% of individuals as an area of incomplete ossification [1, 2]. If present, the foramen is located at the anteroinferior aspect of the EAC, posteromedial to the TMJ. The presence of this foramen may increase the chance of otologic complications during arthroscopy of the TMJ [3]. The cartilaginous and bony portions of the canal are lined with skin containing hairs, sebaceous glands, and ceruminous glands. The adult EAC is approximately 35 mm in length measured from the tip of the tragus to the inferior portion of the tympanic membrane (TM). The diameter of the EAC is approximately 9 mm in the cartilaginous canal and becomes narrower in the bony canal.

The deepest part of the EAC terminates at the TM, which lies obliquely and separates the EAC from the middle ear. The TM has three layers with the outer layer lined by a stratified squamous epithelium and the inner layer lined by a ciliated

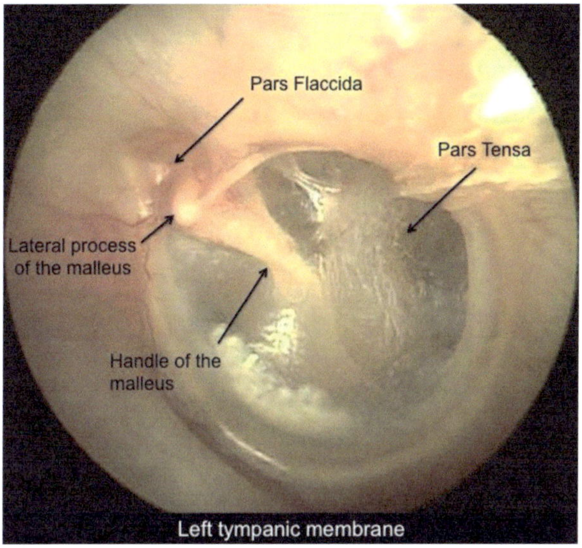

Fig. 4.2 Left tympanic membrane

columnar epithelium with the intervening layer being fibrous. The fibers are attached to the malleus ossicle and also radiate out to the periphery where circumferential fibers are found forming a thickened ring. The TM is divided into the pars tensa and the much smaller pars flaccida superiorly (Fig. 4.2).

Medial to the TM is the middle ear and tympanic cavity, which is lined by ciliated columnar epithelium and connected to the nasopharynx by the Eustachian tube. The tympanic cavity contains the ossicles (malleus, incus, and stapes), the tensor tympani tendon, and the chordae tympani of the facial nerve. The joints between the ossicles are synovial with elastic capsules and supported by several ligaments. Medial to the middle ear, deep in the temporal bone, is the inner ear with its osseous labyrinth of semicircular canals, cochlea, and vestibule.

Violation of the EAC is possible during open joint surgery if regional anatomy is not kept in mind with good spatial awareness on the part of the surgeon. However, perforation/puncture into the EAC and the middle ear is also possible during TMJ arthroscopy. Gonzales reported two cases of EAC puncture in 670 arthroscopies but no TM injuries [4]. Van Sickels reported a case of EAC and middle ear injury after junction of the cartilaginous and bony canal was penetrated [5]. Herzog also reported that a persistent foramen of Huschke might be a risk factor for otologic complications in arthroscopy [3].

Puncture into the cartilaginous portion of the EAC is much more likely, but puncture into the bony portion is possible when using the sharp trocar with excessive force. Once the EAC is entered with the trocar, it is possible to puncture the

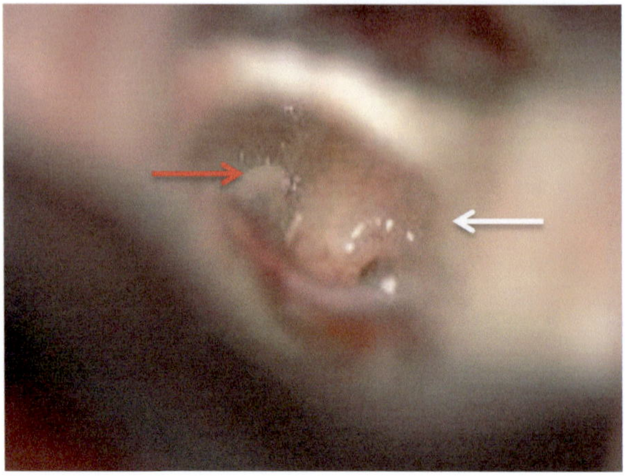

Fig. 4.3 TM puncture from an arthroscope with exposure of the ossicles. *White arrow* TM perforation, *red arrow* stapes

TM and enter the middle ear, causing disruption of the ossicles and hearing loss (Fig. 4.3).

The consequences of puncturing the EAC can vary from minor to serious depending primarily on the location and depth of the puncture. Early recognition of the EAC perforation will often enable the surgeon to redirect instruments and avoid further damage.

4.2.1.1 Potential Sequelae of Puncture into the EAC

Injury isolated to EAC:
- Canal wall laceration and bleeding
- Otitis externa
- Stricture
- Cholesteatoma

Injury involving TM and ossicles:
- Perforation of the TM
- Otitis media
- Otorrhea
- Disruption of the ossicles
- Conductive hearing loss
- Vertigo

4.3 Prevention of the Complication

4.3.1 Open TMJ Surgery

Penetration into the EAC can be avoided during open surgery by careful dissection of soft tissue while being mindful of the EAC proximity, direction, and orientation. The simplest way to avoid this complication is to maintain a plane of dissection anterior to the tragal cartilage down to the postglenoid tubercle. There is the possibility of entering the cartilaginous canal with this approach, but attention should be paid to following the natural angulation of the cartilage. Perforation of the bony canal is also possible particularly when removing bone during bony ankylosis release. In complex bony ankylosis cases, it is sometimes beneficial to utilize navigation surgery to confirm precise anatomic location in relation to surrounding vital structures including the EAC.

4.3.2 Arthroscopic TMJ Surgery

The risk of penetration into the EAC can be minimized during arthroscopic surgery by the use of appropriate force, direction, and precise spatial awareness. The greatest risk is during the initial arthroscopic puncture with the sharp trocar and cannula. McCain reported on a safe, repeatable, and effective puncture technique for single and multiple ports [6]. Tanabe studied and reported the dangerous angles and depths associated with potential middle ear injury during arthroscopy [7].

The risk of inadvertent puncture into the EAC can be minimized by mindful consideration of puncture site, direction, depth, and force.

4.3.2.1 Puncture Site

The more posterior the puncture site, the greater is the risk of EAC perforation. The standard arthroscopic fossa puncture at the peak of the glenoid fossa carries much greater risk than a puncture into the anterior recess.

4.3.2.2 Puncture Direction

The angulation of the trocar upon puncture through the capsule of the TMJ should NOT be perpendicular to the skin, but rather angled anteriorly and directed toward the articular eminence, thereby roughly paralleling the EAC. The trocar should then be angled and directed anterosuperiorly during the puncture (Fig. 4.4).

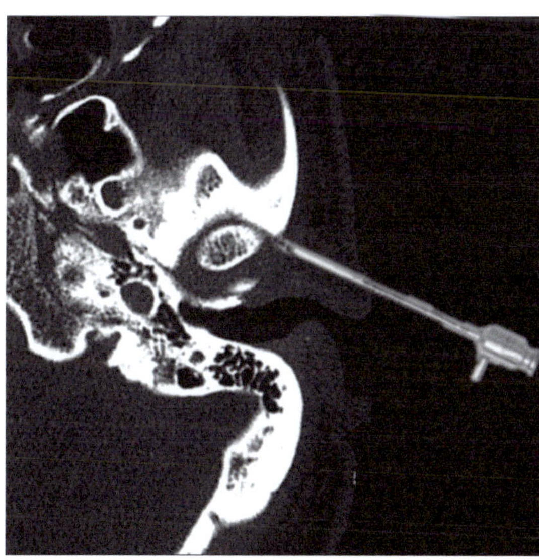

Fig. 4.4 Correct angulation and direction of arthroscopic puncture

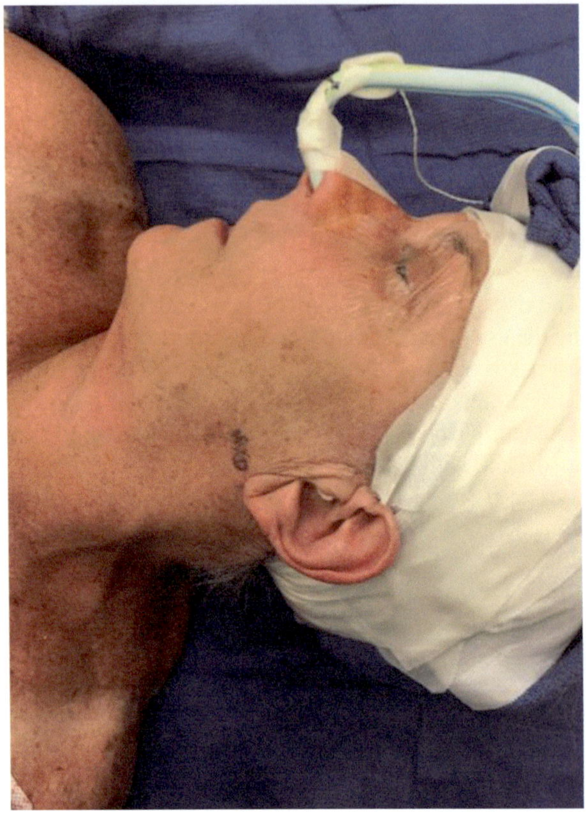

Fig. 4.5 Ideal head position

The position of the patient's head is also critical; the head should be rotated laterally and lay horizontally. Poor head position can result in misdirected punctures due to disorientation of the surgeon (Fig. 4.5).

4.3.2.3 Puncture Depth

The depth of puncture should be 20–25 mm and NEVER greater than 25 mm before removing the sharp trocar, inserting the arthroscope, and confirming position in the joint on the monitor screen. Almost all joints can be entered at this depth, and if the EAC is inadvertently punctured at this depth, the tympanic membrane should not be injured, because it lies at a depth of approximately 35 mm from the tip of the tragal cartilage. Therefore, if the puncture does inadvertently enter into the EAC, the complication will be limited to a laceration in the wall with some bleeding, which is relatively simple to manage.

4.3.2.4 Puncture Force

The puncture force must also be controlled and appropriate. The tenacious lateral capsular ligament creates the most resistance to the trocar puncture. The surgeon must be aware of the resistance to trocar advancement and also when the trocar tip is on bone. This will help to avoid puncture through the bony EAC.

4.4 Recognition and Diagnosis of the Complication

Recognition of penetration into the EAC during TMJ arthroscopy typically occurs when the irrigation line is connected to the cannula and fluid emerges from the ear and EAC or upon initial inspection with the arthroscope while maintaining a safe depth (25 mm), when the normal joint space anatomy is not seen and the tympanic membrane may be seen directly. Although unlikely, it is possible that the TM can be mistaken for a pseudo wall within the joint, so confirmation that the arthroscope is indeed in the joint space is necessary before any mechanical disruption of the pseudo wall is performed.

4.5 Management of the Complication

Once puncture into the EAC is recognized, the extent of injury should immediately be evaluated by detailed otoscopic examination, possibly with the otomicrosope, to determine if the injury is isolated to the EAC wall or if the TM and/or ossicles are also involved. If the surgeon is not comfortable doing this, an otorhinolaryngology (ENT) consultation should be obtained immediately to assist in full evaluation.

4.5.1 Injury Isolated to EAC Wall

If injury to the EAC is limited to a laceration in the wall and minimal bleeding, this can be simply managed by irrigating the EAC with saline (preferably warm to avoid a reflex bradycardia). Persistent bleeding can be managed with Afrin®[1] or oxymetazoline drop instillation into the EAC or judicious cauterization if bleeding persists. Topical ofloxacin otic drop, five drops in the affected ear two times per day for 3–5 days, is recommended. Topical antibiotic combined with steroid otic drops such as ciprofloxacin with dexamethasone, four drops, two times per day for 3–5 days may be used as an alternative. The latter has the potential advantage of the steroid reducing inflammation, granulation tissue, and scar formation.

The EAC laceration may be in the form of a simple puncture or there may be a raised flap of skin. Packing with xeroform gauze, Gelfoam®[2] or ear wick packing can manage skin flaps after the flap has been laid down against the canal wall and will help minimize a hematoma. Packing may be infiltrated with topical antibiotic combined with steroid eardrops. Packing should be removed in 2–3 days at which point the EAC can be reexamined. During healing the EAC should be kept dry to minimize infection. The patient should receive instructions on water precautions (avoiding swimming or any activity where water may enter the ear canal).

It is advisable to obtain an otorhinolaryngology consultation as soon as possible for full evaluation, and an otoscopic examination should be performed at follow-up

[1] ®Bayer, Pittsburgh, PA.

[2] ®Pfizer, New York, NY.

visits to monitor healing. Most lacerations will heal uneventfully, but possible complications include infection, granuloma formation, epithelial inclusion cysts, and strictures. If EAC perforation is recognized and managed intraoperatively in this way, the TMJ arthroscopy can be completed as planned.

4.5.2 Puncture and Perforation of the Tympanic Membrane

If the TM is punctured, it is possible that disruption of the ossicles has also occurred, which can result in significant long-term conductive hearing loss. Disruption of the ossicles requires evaluation and possible surgical repair. If indicated, surgical repair involves repositioning or replacement of the ossicles; the success of which is related to the extent of disruption. Neglected injuries may result in permanent fibrous fixation of the ossicles and significant conductive hearing loss. Therefore, the author recommends an intraoperative otorhinolaryngology consultation, follow-up, and subsequent management of any TM perforation/ossicular disruption. Depending on the severity of the injury, one may consider temporal bone CT without contrast to characterize the extent of injury.

With regard to the tympanic membrane perforation itself, the majority (approximately 80%) of traumatic perforations will heal spontaneously within 4–6 weeks with simple medical management (antibiotic ear drops and water precautions) [8]. Factors that adversely affect the spontaneous healing rate are size of the perforation (>50% area of the TM), older age, and presence of drainage due to infection [9]. Those that fail to heal spontaneously may have consequences dependent on the size and location of the perforation on the TM. These patients may report audible whistling sounds during sneezing and nose blowing, decreased hearing, and a tendency for infection during upper respiratory tract infections and if water enters the ear canal. Perforations are typically not painful unless complicated by infection or cholesteatoma. Perforations in the pars tensa rarely lead to complications, whereas perforations in the pars flaccida carry the longer-term risk of cholesteatoma, and therefore perforations in this location require closer follow-up care.

4.5.3 Initial Medical Management

The goal of initial medical treatment is to control otorrhea, eliminate infection (otitis media), and promote spontaneous healing. Topical ofloxacin otic drop in the affected ear two times per day for 3–5 days for contaminated wounds (e.g., external puncture, perforation with water contamination) is recommended. Topical antibiotic treatment in the presence of a TM perforation carries the risk of ototoxicity, which may result in significant sensorineural hearing loss so it is best to avoid gentamicin, neomycin sulfate, or tobramycin. A combination of ciprofloxacin and dexamethasone otic drops may also be used two times per day for 3–5 days. Systemic antibiotics are required in acute otitis media. Antibiotics (e.g., trimethoprim-sulfamethoxazole or amoxicillin) directed at typical respiratory flora suffice in most cases, but coverage for *Pseudomonas aeruginosa* or resistant *Staphylococcus aureus* may be required.

Water precautions are important and include keeping water out of the ear (avoiding swimming or any activity where water may enter the ear canal). Contaminated water passing through the TM perforation may result in otitis media. This is more likely with large perforations because the surface tension of water limits penetration through small perforations. This may be the reason why there are higher infection rates from hair washing than swimming with small perforations because soap reduces the surface tension of water, facilitating entry through small perforations.

Audiometry is performed after diagnosis and serves as a baseline quantitative evaluation of hearing loss. Audiometry may reveal normal hearing (<25 dB) or a mild conductive loss (26–40 dB) [10]. A significant conductive loss may also indicate ossicular injury and disruption. Patients with TM perforations should be followed and treated by an otolaryngologist. Those that do not heal with medical management may require surgical repair. Indications for surgical repair of persistent non-healing TM perforations include recurrent infections and larger perforations causing hearing loss that affects quality of life [11]. Tympanoplasty to repair a perforation also carries some inherent risk of hearing loss which must be considered [12]. A reasonable alternative to surgery may be a hearing aid device.

4.6 Perforation of the Glenoid Fossa into the Middle Cranial Cavity

4.6.1 Pathophysiology of the Complication

The glenoid or mandibular fossa is a depression in the inferior surface of the squamous part of the temporal bone at the base of the zygomatic process, in which the condyle of the mandible rests. The middle cranial fossa lies directly above and contains the temporal lobe.

The thin roof of the glenoid fossa (GF) separates the joint space from the middle cranial fossa (Figs. 4.6 and 4.7). Cadaveric studies, in which the fossa thickness was

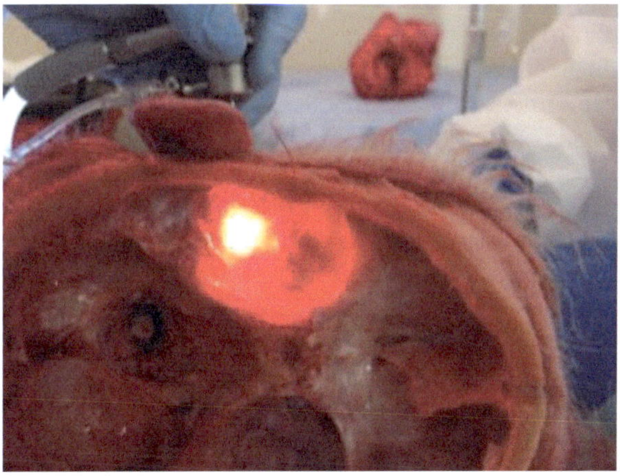

Fig. 4.6 TMJ arthroscopy in a cadaver (cranial vault and brain removed), showing the close relationship between the TMJ and the middle cranial fossa and demonstrating the translucency of the thin glenoid fossa after insertion of the arthroscope

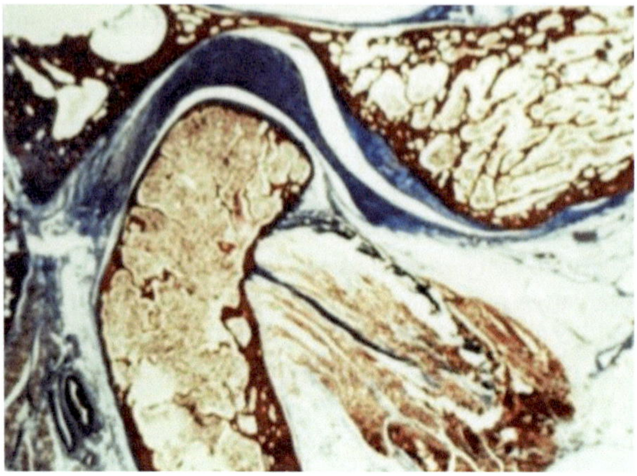

Fig. 4.7 Illustrates the thin roof of the glenoid fossa from a sagittal perspective

measured, show a mean thickness of 0.61 mm with a range of 0.2–1.5 mm in normal joints with intact discs and no osteoarthritis [13, 14]. According to radiographic studies, the GF has been shown to have a mean thickness of 1.22 mm (range 0.5–3 mm) on cone beam computed tomography and a mean thickness of 1.46 mm (0.84–3.57 mm) on magnetic resonance imaging, as it also included thickness of cartilage and periosteum as well as bone [13, 15]. It has also been reported that there may be preexisting anatomic defects in the GF [16].

The intraoperative risk of perforation through the glenoid fossa into the middle cranial fossa is a major concern during both open and arthroscopic surgery. Perforation into the middle cranial fossa has been reported in the literature as a complication of arthroscopic surgery [16–19]. The thin roof of the glenoid fossa can be readily appreciated in a cadaveric specimen undergoing arthroscopy (Fig. 4.6) and with histological specimens (Fig. 4.7).

The risk of injury to the middle cranial fossa contents is rare but has been reported [16, 17, 19–22]. The middle meningeal artery crosses the floor of the middle cranial fossa directly above the roof of the GF, between the bone and the dura. The anterior-posterior distance from the peak height of the glenoid fossa to the middle meningeal artery is on average 2.4 mm (−2 to 8 mm) [23]. Extradural hemorrhage from the middle meningeal artery may occur if the roof of the glenoid fossa is perforated and the artery is injured. Its location within the cranial cavity means that if hemorrhage does occur, it may not be recognized and it is impossible to access from the glenoid fossa. Iatrogenic perforation of the roof of the glenoid fossa can also result in a dural tear and possible exposure of the temporal lobe of the brain resulting in a cerebrospinal fluid (CSF) leak. Arthroscopic irrigation fluid can also enter the middle cranial fossa via a perforation through the roof of the glenoid fossa and may result in symptoms associated with increased intracranial pressure, such as headache, nausea, and vomiting [19]. This can be a difficult to diagnose especially since these symptoms can also be associated with the side effects of general anesthesia (Fig. 4.8).

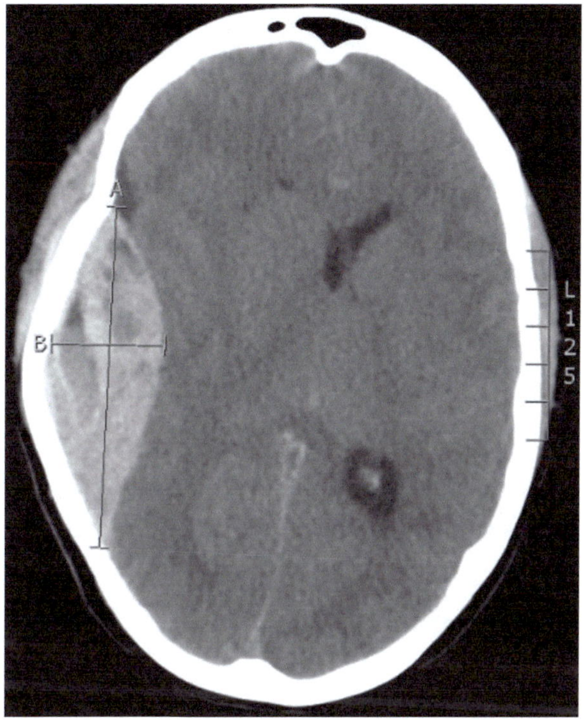

Fig. 4.8 Postoperative extradural hematoma following TMJ arthroscopy. Note the heterogeneous density of the collection, indicating a combination of blood and irrigation fluid

4.6.2 Sequelae of Perforating into the Middle Cranial Fossa

- Arthroscopic irrigation fluid enters the cranial cavity (may be extradural or subdural).
- Bleeding or hemorrhage as a result of injury to the middle meningeal artery.
- Puncture/tear of the dura mater of the temporal lobe.
- Cerebrospinal fluid leakage.
- Extradural or subdural hematoma.
- Injury to the temporal lobe.

4.7 Prevention of the Complication

4.7.1 Open TMJ Surgery

During open TMJ surgery careful surgical dissection is essential to minimize the potential risk of violating the middle cranial fossa. Certain complex surgical cases that involve the joint space, joint ankylosis, or traumatic injury of the fossa can increase the risk of iatrogenic perforation. Careful presurgical workup with a preoperative CT or MRI scan has become standard and can help in identifying areas that would be of concern in patients with erosive changes, joint ankylosis, or tumors. The use of virtual surgical planning or navigation surgery along with surgical precision can help to minimize the risk of violating the middle cranial fossa during dissection and bone removal in and around the glenoid fossa.

4.7.2 Arthroscopic TMJ Surgery

During arthroscopic surgery, it is important to be aware of angulation as well as depth of the instruments at all times. Directing the instruments toward the articular eminence and not toward the glenoid fossa can prevent complications associated with perforation of the roof of the glenoid fossa. As discussed in the earlier part of the chapter, close attention needs to be directed to puncture site, direction, depth, and force.

4.7.2.1 Puncture Site

Puncture sites in and around the peak height of the glenoid fossa carry greater risk of GF perforation.

4.7.2.2 Puncture Direction

The angulation and direction of the trocar upon puncture through the capsule of the TMJ should be directed carefully with a slight upward direction to avoid the disc, but it should NOT be directed toward the GF. The position of the patient's head is again important and should be as described earlier. Again, poor head position can result in misdirected punctures due to disorientation of the surgeon.

4.7.2.3 Puncture Depth

Maintaining the depth of initial puncture at 20–25 mm will not avoid perforation of the GF if the trocar is directed toward it.

4.7.2.4 Puncture Force

The puncture force must also be controlled and appropriate. The tenacious lateral capsular ligament creates the most resistance to the trocar puncture. Once the joint space is entered, manipulation should be with delicate and gentle force, and the sharp trocar should be removed. The surgeon must again be aware of the resistance to trocar advancement and also when the trocar tip is on the bone.

4.8 Recognition and Diagnosis of the Complication

During both open and arthroscopic surgeries, the GF perforation may be directly visualized during surgery. However, small perforations may be missed and even concealed by the fibrocartilage lining the fossa, in which case, the symptoms associated with perforation into the middle cranial fossa may present in the immediate postoperative period. Complaints of a headache, nausea, vomiting, vertigo, and palsies of the cranial nerves of the ipsilateral side are all associated with raised intracranial pressure and should be recognized. Delayed bleeding or a hematoma within the intracranial fossa can be difficult to detect, and signs such as headache, irritability, nausea or vomiting, and change in behavior should be considered an indication of cerebral irritation. If there is a suspicion of GF perforation, a head CT without contrast should be obtained immediately.

Arthroscopic irrigation fluid within the cranial cavity can also cause symptoms associated with increased intracranial pressure and cerebral irritation that is self-limiting. Physiological reabsorption of the fluid leads to an eventual reduction in pressure and resolution of the symptoms. However, close monitoring of vital parameters including ICP measurement and cranial nerve function is necessary.

4.9 Management of the Complication

A perforation in the roof of the glenoid fossa during open or arthroscopic TMJ surgery may result in isolated bony injury/perforation, bleeding from the middle meningeal vessels, dural tear and CSF leak, and injury to the temporal lobe itself.

Upon recognition of a perforation through the roof of the GF, it is essential to obtain an immediate neurosurgery consultation and evaluation. The evaluation should determine if the perforation is an isolated injury to the bone only or if it is associated with bleeding from the middle meningeal vessels or even a dural tear with CSF leak. This may necessitate immediate neurosurgical intervention.

During open TMJ surgery, a CSF leak through the roof of the glenoid fossa perforation is readily recognizable, but with arthroscopic surgery, this is not possible because of the continuous fluid flow used during arthroscopic surgery. Intracranial bleeding is the most pressing complication to recognize and manage because this may result in sudden and progressive increase in intracranial pressure (ICP), brain compression, and even herniation or death.

If the dura is intact, any bleeding from the middle meningeal vessels will result in an extradural hemorrhage/hematoma, as opposed to a subdural hemorrhage if the dura is also perforated or torn. A baseline head CT without contrast should be obtained in all cases. As in trauma protocols, the CT is repeated at 6–8 h to identify any interval change and assess the stability of any hematoma, which will determine the need for additional interventions, such as an intraventricular catheter (IVC) placement, a lumbar drain placement, or a craniotomy. These additional interventions also may be indicated if there is a change in the vital signs and neurologic status of the patient during the monitoring phase. Intraventricular catheter placement allows both ICP monitoring and also the ability to drain CSF, thereby reducing the ICP, and may also be useful in the setting of a CSF leak. A normal ICP ranges from 1 to 20 mmHg.

4.9.1 Bone Perforation Only

Immediate neurosurgery consult is advisable to carefully investigate whether there is any violation of the dura or CSF leak (open surgery). A baseline CT without contrast to exclude an intracranial bleed is warranted. A robust neurosurgical monitoring protocol to monitor neurological status may be needed. Consider a repeat CT without contrast after 6 h if there are neurological changes during monitoring. Postoperative antibiotics are usually not needed if there is no dural tear.

4.9.2 Bleeding and Extradural/Subdural Hematoma

This mandates an immediate neurosurgery consult, baseline CT scan, and neurological monitoring in a dedicated neurosurgery ICU setting. Neurosurgical intervention or repeat CT without contrast may be required. Antibiotics may also be indicated.

4.9.3 Dural Tear and CSF Leak

If the dural tear is small, it may be possible to seal the leak with fibrin glue and local hemostatic agents. Neurosurgical consultation is recommended as an IVC or lumbar drain may be needed. A baseline noncontrast CT to exclude intracranial bleeding, dedicated neurosurgical monitoring in an ICU setting, and antibiotics are also needed.

References

1. Lacout A, Marsot-Dupuch K, WRK S, Lasjaunias P. Foramen tympanicum, or foramen of Huschke: pathologic cases and anatomic CT study. Am J Neuroradiol. 2005;26(6):1317–23.
2. Tozoğlu U, Caglayan F, Harorli A. Foramen tympanicum or foramen of Huschke: anatomical cone beam CT study. Dentomaxillofac Radiol. 2012;41(4):294–7.
3. Herzog S, Fiese R. Persistent foramen of Huschke: possible risk factor for otologic complications after arthroscopy of the temporomandibular joint. Oral Surg Oral Med Oral Pathol. 1989;68(3):267–70.
4. Gonzalez-Garcia R, Rodriguez-Campo FJ, Escorial-Hernandez V, et al. Complications of temporomandibular joint arthroscopy: a Retrospective Analytic Study of 670 Arthroscopic Procedures. J Oral Maxillofac Surg. 2006;64(11):1587–91.
5. Van Sickels JE, Nishioka GJ, Hegewald MD, Neal GD. Middle ear injury resulting from temporomandibular joint arthroscopy. J Oral Maxillofac Surg. 1987;45(11):962–5.
6. McCain JP, de la Rua H, LeBlanc WG. Puncture technique and portals of entry for diagnostic and operative arthroscopy of the temporomandibular joint. Arthrosc J Arthrosc Relat Surg. 1991;7(2):221–32.
7. Sugisaki M, Ikai A, Tanabe H. Dangerous angles and depths for middle ear and middle cranial fossa injury during arthroscopy of the temporomandibular joint. J Oral Maxillofac Surg. 1995;53(7):803–10.
8. Kristensen S. Spontaneous healing of traumatic tympanic membrane perforations in man: a century of experience. J Laryngol Otol. 1992;106(12):1037–50.
9. Orji FT, Agu CC. Determinants of spontaneous healing in traumatic perforations of the tympanic membrane. Clin Otolaryngol. 2008;33(5):420–6.
10. Couch ME. Cummings otolaryngology. In: Head and neck surgery. Philadelphia: Elsevier; 2010.
11. Lerut B, Pfammatter A, Moons J, Linder T. Functional correlations of tympanic membrane perforation size. Otol Neurotol. 2012;33(3):379–86.

12. Röösli C, Sim JH, Chatzimichalis M, Huber AM. How does closure of tympanic membrane perforations affect hearing and middle ear mechanics? – An evaluation in a patient cohort and temporal bone models. Otol Neurotol. 2012;33(3):371–8.
13. Honda K, Arai Y, Kashima M, et al. Evaluation of the usefulness of the limited cone-beam CT (3DX) in the assessment of the thickness of the roof of the glenoid fossa of the temporomandibular joint. Dentomaxillofac Radiol. 2004;33(6):391–5.
14. Holmlund A, Hellsing G. Arthroscopy of the temporomandibular joint. An autopsy study. Int J Oral Surg. 1985;14(2):169–75.
15. Perrott DH, Alborzi A, Kaban LB, Helms CA. A prospective evaluation of the effectiveness of temporomandibular joint arthroscopy. J Oral Maxillofac Surg. 1990;48(10):1029–32.
16. Murphy MA, Silvester KC, Chan TY. Extradural haematoma after temporomandibular joint arthroscopy. A case report. Int J Oral Maxillofac Surg. 1993;22(6):332–5.
17. JP MC. Arthroscopy of the human temporomandibular joint. J Oral Maxillofac Surg. 1988;46(8):648–55.
18. Carter JB. Complications of TMJ arthroscopy: a review of 2,225 cases. J Oral Maxillofac Surg. 1988;46(12):M14–5.
19. Patel S, Jerjes W, Upile T, Hopper C. Short communication TMJ arthroscopy: rare neurological complications associated with breach of the skull base. Br J Oral Maxillofac Surg. 2010;48(4):e18–20.
20. Greene MW, Hackney FL, Van Sickels JE. Arthroscopy of the temporomandibular joint: an anatomic perspective. J Oral Maxillofac Surg. 1989;47(4):386–9.
21. Greene MW, van Sickels JE. Survey of TMJ arthroscopy in oral and maxillofacial surgery residency programs. J Oral Maxillofac Surg. 1989;47(6):574–6.
22. Westesson PL, Eriksson L, Liedberg J. The risk of damage to facial nerve, superficial temporal vessels, disk, and articular surfaces during arthroscopic examination of the temporomandibular joint. Oral Surg Oral Med Oral Pathol. 1986;62(2):124–7.
23. Talebzadeh N, Rosenstein TP, Pogrel MA. Anatomy of the structures medial to the temporomandibular joint. Oral Surg Oral Med Oral Pathol Oral Radiol Endod. 1999;88(6):674–8.

Facial Nerve Injury

5

Hany Emam, Courtney Jatana, and Gregory M. Ness

5.1 Introduction

Minimizing risk to the integrity of the facial nerve is a critical measure of surgical success in temporomandibular joint (TMJ) surgeries. The surgeon must have a keen understanding of the regional anatomy combined with a planned dissection to protect the facial nerve in their approach to the joint [1]. Facial nerve injury may have devastating effects on the patient esthetically and functionally due to impairment of the frontalis and/or orbicularis oculi muscles. According to Liu et al., the most current review of the literature reveals that the incidence of facial nerve injury in conjunction with open TMJ surgery ranges from 12.5 to 32% [2]. The chapter will provide a review on the anatomy of the facial nerve, procedures leading to potential injury, recognition of injury, and multiple methods of management.

5.2 Pathophysiology

The course of the facial nerve and its branches (Fig. 5.1) must be known to avoid violating the boundaries of safe surgery and creating a potentially paralyzing injury. The temporal and zygomatic branches of the facial nerve are most at risk of injury in TMJ surgery. These two branches of the facial nerve are situated deep to the superficial temporal fascia and superficial to the superficial layer of the deep temporal fascia and periosteum, overlying the root of the zygoma. (Fig. 5.2). In their landmark 1979 article, Al-Kayat and Bramley measured the location of the facial nerve's main trunk and found that it runs no nearer than 1.5 cm below the inferior margin of the bony external auditory meatus. The temporal branch of the nerve crosses the zygomatic

H. Emam, BDS, MS • C. Jatana, DDS, MS, FACS • G.M. Ness, DDS, FACS (✉)
Division of Oral and Maxillofacial Surgery & Dental Anesthesiology, The Ohio State University College of Dentistry, Columbus, OH, USA
e-mail: ness.8@osu.edu

G.F. Bouloux (ed.), *Complications of Temporomandibular Joint Surgery*,
DOI 10.1007/978-3-319-51241-9_5

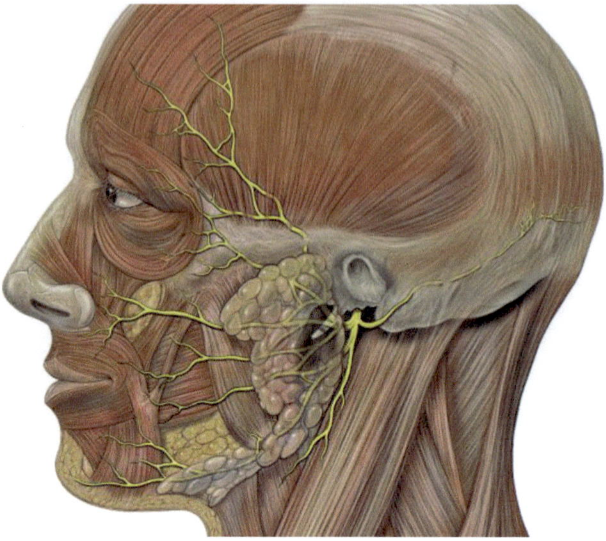

Fig. 5.1 Facial nerve branches (Adapted from Ness [3]; with permission – Courtesy of Patrick J. Lynch, medical illustrator; C. Carl Jaffe, MD, cardiologist, Yale University School of Medicine, Center for Advanced Instructional Media, New Haven, CT. Published under Creative Commons Attribution 2.5 License 2006)

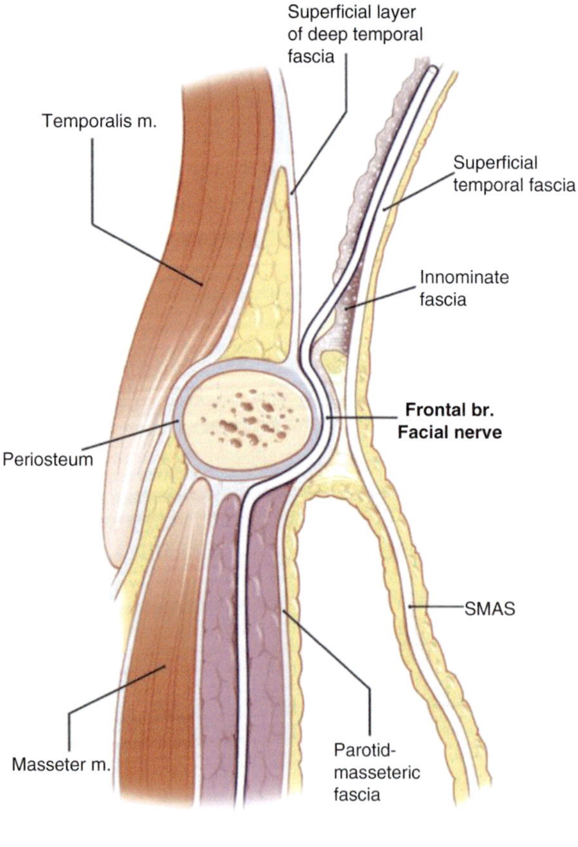

Fig. 5.2 Frontal diagram showing the tissue planes superficial and slightly anterior to the TMJ. The central bony structure is the cut end of the zygomatic arch (Adapted from Ness [3]; with permission – From Agarwal, et al. [4])

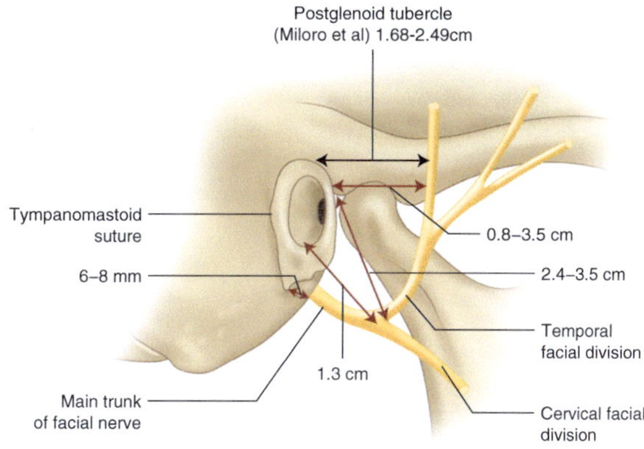

Fig. 5.3 Distance between the external auditory canal and temporal (frontal) branch of the facial nerve (Adapted from Ness [3]; with permission – Miloro, et al. [6])

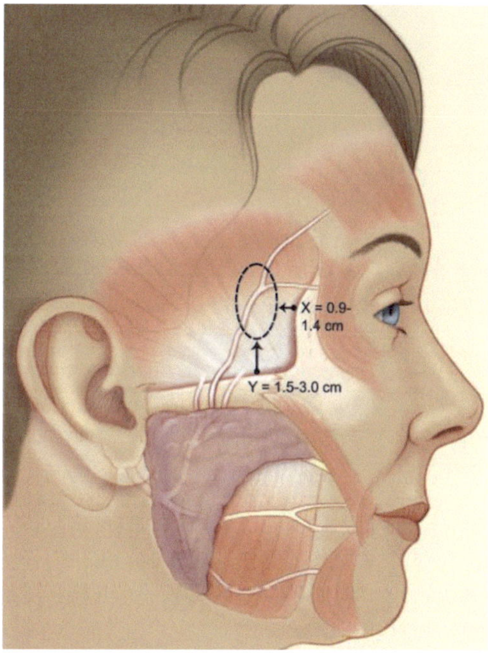

Fig. 5.4 Area in which the temporal (frontal) branch of the facial nerve transitions from lying deep in the superficial temporal fascia to piercing it from below (Adapted from Ness [3]; with permission – Agarwal, et al. [4])

arch at a minimum distance of 0.8 cm and a mean of 2.0 cm anterior to the bony external auditory meatus. Similar cadaver studies by Woltmann found a minimum distance of 0.7 cm and a mean of 1.5 cm, whereas a high-resolution MRI study of live subjects by Miloro and others measured a minimum distance of 1.7 cm and a mean of 2.1 cm (Fig. 5.3). Agarwal and others have further increased our knowledge of the facial nerve's path in three dimensions. They showed that the temporal branch lies in the loose areolar connective tissue layer between the superficial and deep temporal fascia as it crosses the zygomatic arch before entering the superficial temporal fascia from its undersurface in a consistent region 1.5. to 3.0 cm above the zygomatic arch and 0.9 to 1.4 cm posterior to the lateral orbital rim [3–7] (Fig. 5.4).

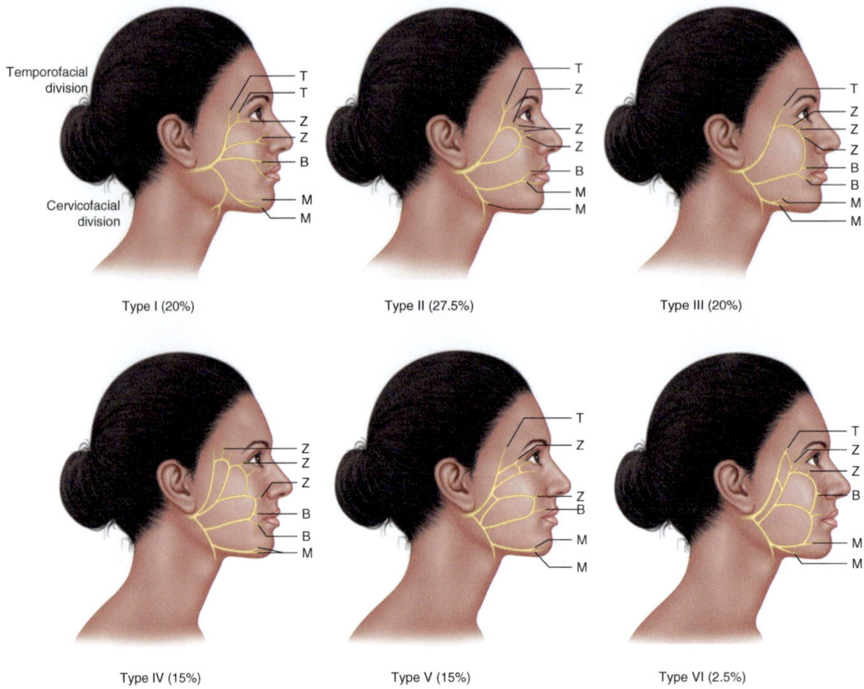

Fig. 5.5 Terminal branches of the facial nerve, demonstrating its variability. *B* buccal, *M* mandibular, *T* temporal, *Z* zygomatic (Adapted from Callander [8])

The TMJ surgeon should also be aware of the variability of the terminal branches: temporal, zygomatic, buccal, mandibular, and cervical. In another landmark study performed with 100 cadaver heads, there were eight variations in the distribution of the facial nerve. Of surgical significance, the author found distal branching of the temporal branch in four separate patterns [8]. This variation allows for several pathways to innervate the frontalis muscle. Hall et al. found that the most distal branching of the facial nerve occurs 63% of the time. With this common pattern, the temporal branch can be injured without losing frontalis function [9] (Fig. 5.5).

5.3 TMJ Procedures and Risk for Facial Nerve Injury

5.3.1 Arthrocentesis and Arthroscopy

The anatomical locations of the entry and exit points for either arthrocentesis or arthroscopy are designed to avoid injury to the facial nerve with needle puncture. These locations were developed and described in the literature by Westesson et al. and Holmlund and Hellsing. Descriptively, the first entry puncture point is located

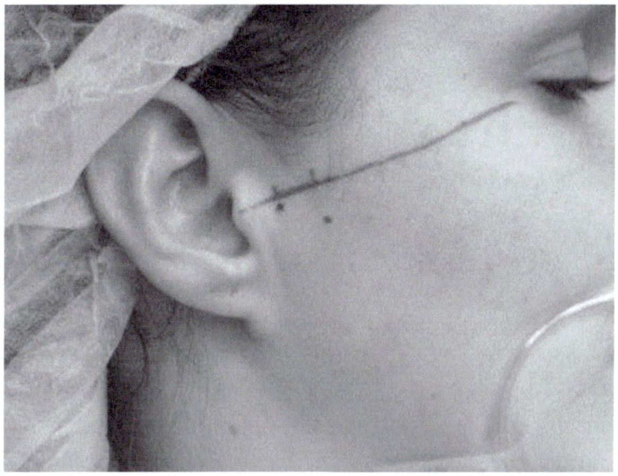

Fig. 5.6 Drawing of the entry and exit ports for arthrocentesis/arthroscopy

Table 5.1 Possible causes of facial nerve injury in arthrocentesis and arthroscopy

Failure to use standard anatomic landmarks
Local anesthesia inadvertently injected
Poor flow of outflow leading to hydrostatic pressure
Inadvertent movement of the scope through the medial capsule; fluid compression into pterygomandibular space
Inappropriate usage of electrocautery
Stretching of tissue due to improper instrumentation usage

10 mm anterior to the tragus and 2 mm inferior to the tragal-canthal line, while the second port site is 20 mm anterior to the tragus and 10 mm inferior to the tragal-canthal line [10, 11] (Fig. 5.6).

Potential sources of facial nerve injury during arthrocentesis and/or arthroscopy include incorrect placement or excessive attempts at placing ports. Poor outflow of fluid can lead to increased hydrostatic pressure within the joint space risking possible compression injury on the nerve. Arthroscopy, due to the invasive nature of the procedure, has more specific risks than arthrocentesis. Instrumentation injuries such as stretching of soft tissues, perforation of the medial capsule allowing fluid into the pterygomandibular space, and/or trauma from electrocautery can be damaging to the nerve. In general, with arthrocentesis and/or arthroscopy, the facial nerve may be injured from compression, tension, and stretching, although the incidence of permanent injury is rare [2] (Table 5.1).

5.3.2 Open TMJ Procedures

Dissection to the temporomandibular joint by any preferred approach could potentially lead to facial nerve injury. Maintaining the correct fascial plane is critical to protecting the nerve. Surgery on a multiply operated joint is potentially problematic

Table 5.2 Possible causes of facial nerve injury in open TMJ surgery

Local anesthesia inadvertently injected
Excessive retraction and/or traction
Thermal injury from electrocautery
Crushing by forceps or clamps
Incorrect placement of vascular clips
Incorrect placement of plication sutures
Hematoma or edema in the nerve sheath
Inflammation and/or infection

in that tissue planes are poorly defined and the facial nerve may be surrounded by dense scar tissue. Dissection and identification of the correct fascial plane can then be challenging, increasing the potential for nerve injury. Excessive retraction for visualization can pull the fascia and lead to either compression and/or stretching injuries of nerve fibers. The use of electrocautery during the procedure as well as crushing or clamping of tissue with instruments due to bleeding can also injure the facial nerve. Precise closure must be done as inadvertent placement of the suture needle could potentially damage the nerve. Postoperative swelling and/or hematoma formation can also lead to a compression injury; therefore, it is wise to obtain hemostasis and use a pressure dressing following surgery [2] (Table 5.2).

5.4 Prevention of the Facial Nerve Injury

5.4.1 Facial Nerve Monitoring

Facial nerve monitoring has been a standard of practice for head and neck surgeons since the 1980s in order to minimize and prevent facial nerve injury. Monitoring can be defined into either "passive" or "active" forms. In the passive form, facial muscle movement is activated only by direct mechanical, stretch, or other nonelectrical stimulation of the facial nerve. As the simplest example, having a resident or a surgical assistant visually monitoring the face for twitching during a surgical approach to the TMJ is the simplest form of passive monitoring. A handheld device with a tip carrying low amplitude impulses to tissue in order to stimulate any nearby branch of the facial nerve is a common device applying passive monitoring in most TMJ surgeon's practices. In the most advanced form of passive monitoring, electrodes placed near the orbicularis oculi and orbicularis oris muscles record electromyography (EMG) potentials that are audible to the surgeon when he or she approaches or encroaches on a branch of the facial nerve [12].

In active monitoring, the facial nerve itself is electrically stimulated with audible recordings of facial compound muscle action potentials (CAMP). The stimulation is delivered through either a monopolar or bipolar electrode with blunt tips. On bipolar stimulation, the current is confined to the tissue between the electrified tips allowing for a very specific stimulation. The same stimulus is created using monopolar tips, but it does not identify the nerve location with the same specificity [12].

These techniques are not fool proof and failure to stimulate the facial nerve could be from many sources including detached or incorrectly placed electrodes, a malfunction of the handheld stimulator, infiltration from local anesthetic paralyzing the nerve, pharmacological muscular paralysis from the induction of anesthesia, and even a muted speaker. Attempts should be made to avoid these errors by intraoperative checks of the monitor, communicating with the anesthesiologist, and being competent in the surgical anatomy and approach to the temporomandibular joint [12].

5.4.2 Surgical Approaches to the TMJ to Avoid Facial Nerve Injury

There are several incisions for approaching the TMJ. The difficulty with any approach is the ability to provide for adequate exposure without injuring the facial nerve. The preauricular incision is most commonly used. In this approach, the skin incision line is drawn (Fig. 5.7) by making use of any previous incision scars or strategically located fine skin wrinkles. Once the skin incision is made, the avascular plane immediately anterior to the perichondrium of the external

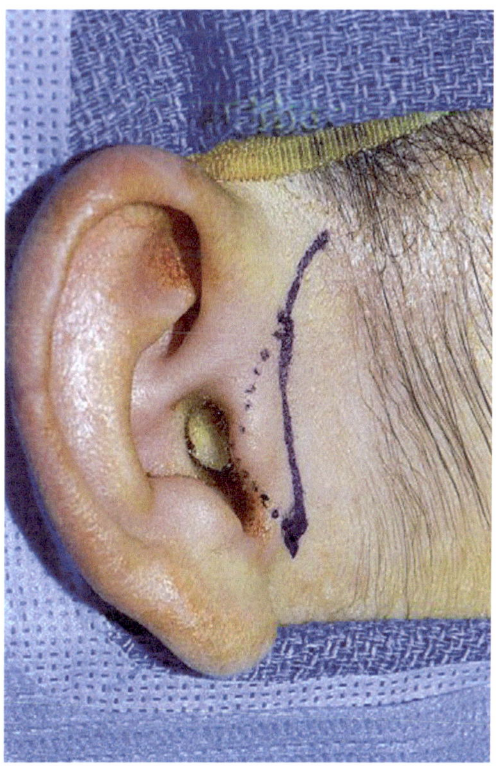

Fig. 5.7 Preauricular skin incision line. Many surgeons prefer an endaural incision placed at variable distances posterior to the dotted line where it is less visible (Adapted from Ness [3]; with permission)

auditory canal wall's anterior surface is opened bluntly, beginning just deep to the skin at the base of the tragus. Once the cartilage surface is located, the dissection must be directed medially and anteriorly, not perpendicular to the skin surface, to follow the path of the auditory canal cartilage and avoid injury to the ear. When in the correct plane, this initial dissection creates a clean, bloodless pocket immediately anterior to the tragus that ends bluntly at the depth of the parotidomasseteric fascia. Dissection continues through the superficial temporal fascia until the smooth, white, well-defined surface of the deep temporal fascia is exposed. Dissection continues deeply until the zygomatic arch is palpable under the superficial layer of the deep temporal fascia, which divides 1–2 cm above the arch to surround it. The tissues anterior and superficial to this plane are retracted gently to minimize any traction on the temporal branch of the facial nerve, and only a narrow band of the fascia over the zygomatic arch is exposed just superior to the auditory canal cartilage and connecting the two initial dissections. A scalpel blade is then used to make an incision in the superficial layer of the deep temporal fascia in the same plane as the dissection to expose the area, beginning about 1 cm above the zygomatic arch. The incision is then extended inferiorly across the zygomatic arch, and then a periosteal elevator is used to dissect under the superficial layer of the deep temporal fascia; retracting from beneath this layer protects and retracts branches of the facial nerve. The overall goal of this approach is to dissect and elevate a continuous layer from superior to inferior containing the temporal fascia, the superficial layer of the temporal fascia, and the periosteum to prevent injury to the nerve [3].

Modifications of this technique have been described. A deep subfascial approach offers an additional protective layer for the facial nerve (the deep layer of the deep temporalis fascia and temporal fat pad). In comparison to the traditional technique described above, the incision of the upper and lower layer of the deep temporalis fascia is completely through the fat tissue, exposing the fibers of the temporal muscle and producing this subfascial layer (under the deep temporal fascia) [13].

5.5 Recognition and Diagnosis

Dysfunction of the facial nerve can result in several undesirable effects. Clinical consequences from injury may cause either a defect in facial expression or a functional deficit and/or may leave the patient with a cosmetic deformity all of which may lead to psychosocial issues. Studies have shown the incidence of facial nerve injury following TMJ surgery ranges from 12.5 to 32%. The majority of these injuries tend to be temporary with full return to function within 2–6 months [14].

The surgeon should evaluate all patients for facial nerve injury in the postoperative setting. A thorough clinical exam should be performed and any injury documented. Since weakness can be subtle, it helps to compare the operated side to the non-operated side when surgery is unilateral. There are specific clinical findings that will be associated depending on which terminal nerve branch is

Table 5.3 Terminal branches and the action on the corresponding facial muscle

Muscle	Facial nerve branch	Action
Corrugator supercilii Procerus	Temporal	Pulls the eyebrow medially and downward Pulls the medial eyebrow downward
Orbicularis oculi Zygomatic major	Temporal and zygomatic Zygomatic and buccal	Closes the eyelid and contracts the skin around the eye Elevates corners of the mouth
Zygomaticus minor Levator labii superioris Risorius Buccinator Orbicularis oris Levator labii superioris alaeque nasi	Buccal	Elevates the upper lip Elevates the upper lip and midportion nasolabial fold Aids smile with lateral pull Pulls corner of the mouth backward and compresses the cheek Closes and compresses the lips Elevates the medial nasolabial fold and nasal ala
Depressor anguli oris Depressor labii inferioris Mentalis	Buccal and marginal mandibular Marginal mandibular	Pulls corners of the mouth downward Pulls down the lower lip Pulls the skin of the chin upward
Platysma	Cervical	Pulls down corners of the mouth

injured and what muscle is innervated (Table 5.3). Observation of any difficulty or inability in the patient to raise their affected eyebrow, wrinkle their forehead, completely close their eyelids (lagophthalmos), and/or smile symmetrically could signify a facial nerve injury. There may also be limitations or dysfunction to special functions such as lacrimation, salivation, and taste. Particularly with lagophthalmos, lack of treatment can lead to exposure keratitis, corneal ulceration, and blindness.

If there is clinical injury, classifying the degree and type of nerve lesion becomes important, particularly for prognosis and planning treatment. There is no "gold standard" method of grading these injuries due to the subjectivity of assessment and reporting. Attempts have been made to develop a universal objective measurement, ranging from a simple diagnosis with handheld calipers to using complex processes with digital photographic and videographic computer systems. Several classification systems have been devised, but since the 1980s, the House-Brackmann system has been the most widely accepted system [12, 15–17]. There are six grades to this system, with grade I indicating normal function of the facial nerve and grade VI indicating total paralysis. The system is limited by ambiguity to distinguish accurately among the finer grades of dysfunction [12] (Table 5.4).

In addition to clinical classification of facial nerve injury with the House-Brackmann grading scale, understanding the use of electrical musculature testing is helpful in diagnosing and future treatment of the nerve injury. The goal of electrodiagnostic testing is to help evaluate the degree of facial nerve injury and the functionality of the facial musculature. Commonly used electrical tests are the nerve

Table 5.4 House-Brackmann facial nerve injury grading system

Grade	Description	Characteristics
I	Normal	Normal facial function
II	Mild	*At rest*: Normal symmetry and tone *Forehead motion*: Moderate to good *Eye motion*: Compete closure with minimum effort *Mouth motion*: Slight asymmetry
III	Moderate	*At rest*: Normal symmetry and tone *Forehead motion*: Slight to moderate *Eye motion*: Compete closure with effort *Mouth motion*: Slightly weak with maximum effort
IV	Moderately severe	*At rest*: Normal symmetry and tone *Forehead motion*: None *Eye motion*: Incomplete closure *Mouth motion*: Asymmetric with maximum effort
V	Severe	*At rest*: Asymmetry *Forehead motion*: None *Eye motion*: Incomplete closure *Mouth motion*: Slight movement
VI	Total paralysis	No movement

excitability test (NET), maximum stimulation test (MST), electroneurography (ENoG), and electromyography (EMG) [12, 18]:

1. *Nerve excitability threshold* (*NET*): Requires a Hilger nerve stimulator, with the extratemporal portion of the nerve stimulated with a small, pulsed DC current. The face is observed for the lowest current to produce a visible twitch.
2. *Maximal stimulation test* (*MST*): Is a modified version of the NET, with an attempt to determine the difference between the strength and amount of contraction. Allows for interobserver variation.
3. *Electroneurography* (*ENoG*): This exam adds the ability to record facial muscle action potential with surface or needled electrodes to the stimulation tests. Percentages based on compound action potential (CAP) are used for interpretation. Excellent recovery of facial function occurs when the CAP in ENoG does not reach 90%.
4. *Electromyography* (*EMG*): Measures muscle action potential generated by spontaneous and voluntary action. Researchers have found that EMG had 80% accuracy in predicting a poor outcome 10–14 days after onset of paralysis.

Currently, there is no standard of care when to use nonoperative vs. operative management with electrodiagnostic testing. Research has shown surgical exploration is warranted when ENoG tests produce an amplitude ratio > 90%; NET shows a difference of 3.5 mA or the MST shows no reaction when combined with EMG. Electromyography alone provides important information that can also help determine treatment options. Typically, resting muscle exhibits no spontaneous electrical activity. In the setting of denervation from nerve injury, electrical activity may be increased, and spontaneous fibrillation potentials develop. These fibrillation potentials are strong evidence that denervation has occurred and may encourage the surgeon to surgically explore.

In combination with electrodiagnostic testing, understanding the Sunderland classification is an additional helpful tool that uses a histopathological description of the nerve injury when deciding whether surgical exploration or management is necessary. There are five classes to this system that are listed as follows:

Class I: There is no physical disruption of axonal continuity with supportive tissue elements remain intact.

Class II: Generally caused by pressure, will have axonal disruption without injury to supporting structures. Wallerian degeneration occurs and propagates distally from site of injury.

Class III: Endoneurium disruption occurs and Wallerian degeneration occurs similar to Class II.

Class IV: Perineural disruption, implying a more severe injury and potential for incomplete or aberrant regeneration is common.

Class V: Complete transection of the facial nerve, including epineural sheath, carries almost no hope for useful regeneration.

5.5.1 There are important clinical findings to these classes in relation to electrodiagnostic testing. When a Class I injury has occurred, the facial muscles cannot be moved voluntarily, but a facial twitch can be elicited by electrodiagnostic testing of the nerve distal to the site of injury. This is helpful to understand the nerve may not need surgical exploration with this result. Class II to V injuries will involve some form of axonal discontinuity. In these injuries, electrodiagnostic testing will fail to produce a propagated action potential and muscle contraction within 1 week. In the case of facial nerve injury, the delay in Wallerian degeneration results in continued electrical stimulation of the distal segment for 3–5 days. It is important to note that during these first few days after an insult, electrodiagnostic testing of any form cannot distinguish between the various classes of injuries [12, 18].

5.6 Management of Facial Nerve Injury

After a complete physical examination is performed in addition to classifying the degree of injury by electrodiagnostic testing, the surgeon is faced with the decision of when and how to proceed with facial reanimation. The complex decision must also include considerations of patient-specific factors such as age, medical status, skin type, motivation for rehabilitation, and likelihood of appropriate

Table 5.5 Common surgical techniques

Surgical treatment options for facial nerve injury
Primary nerve repair
Cross-face grafting
Cable grafting
Regional muscle transposition
Free muscle flaps
Hypoglossal-facial nerve transfer
Static facial procedures: For example, upper lid gold weight, browlift, blepharoplasty, sling, and lower lid procedures

follow-up. Rehabilitation of the patient with facial nerve injury can include a comprehensive program that includes medical management, physiotherapy, psychosocial support, and the possibility of a myriad of surgical procedures available [19, 20] (Table 5.5).

5.6.1 Nonsurgical Techniques

In cases where the facial nerve is thought to be intact, nonsurgical management is best. These patients should be observed from 6 months to 2 years. Injuries to the temporal and/or zygomatic branches typically are not directly visualized nerve injuries, which make the clinical decision more challenging to manage. If nonsurgical management is chosen, the conservative palliative options include physiotherapy, exercises, and reassurance. Physical therapy is often underutilized in the setting of facial nerve injury [21]. Facial neuromuscular reeducation using surface EMG and biofeedback techniques have demonstrated improvements in facial movement in randomized trials. Botox and corrective makeup techniques have also been used in management of the reanimation of the facial muscles [19]. Types of nonsurgical management are as follows:

1. Medical management
   The primary goal is to protect the cornea from sight-threatening complications. Correction of eyelid malposition, reduction of epiphora, and improvement of cosmetic concerns are therefore secondary goals. Corneal protection begins with a regimen of regular ocular lubrication and, at minimum, should include application of artificial tears five to ten times per day with ophthalmic ointment at night. Other supplemental measures include the usage of a moisture chamber and taping [22].
2. Physical therapy
   Methods of rehabilitation for facial paralysis have included massage, electrical stimulation, and repetition of common facial expressions. The most promising treatment technique is facial neuromuscular reeducation using

surface electromyography (sEMG) or mirror biofeedback. This is a process of relearning facial movement using specific and accurate feedback to enhance facial muscle activity while suppressing abnormal movement. The program is highly individualized and requires multiple visits to a physical therapist for treatment. Any of these techniques should be considered early in the evaluation of facial nerve injury and implemented immediately for positive results [15, 23, 24].

3. Botulinum toxin
   Botox is a relatively new treatment in the nonsurgical armamentarium for management of facial nerve injuries. In the context of facial neuromuscular disorders, Botox was initially used to treat patients with symptoms due to Bell's palsy. When the facial nerve is injured in the approach to the temporomandibular joint, possible aberrant regeneration of fibers may lead to unwanted affects such as involuntary spasms of the orbicularis oculi and lacrimation of the affected eye (synkinesis). Botox works by blocking the presynaptic release of acetylcholine, which causes functional denervation of neuromuscular endplates. Because fibers to the lacrimal gland utilize acetylcholine as a neurotransmitter, local injections of Botox into the gland can remedy lacrimation. Injection into the orbicularis oculi muscle can control facial synkinesis.
   Botox may also be applied to the non-operated (contralateral) frontalis muscle to mask the operated (ipsilateral) frontalis weakness [15, 25, 26].
4. Corrective makeup techniques
   Outside of the typical use of covering one's face for color, makeup can be used as a cognitive interactive technique that can change a person's appearance and create different impressions using optical illusions. Kanzaki et al. reported the use of makeup techniques to improve the appearance in two women with House-Brackmann grade III. An expert beautician instructed the women on the application of makeup to correct facial imbalance. In both cases, it was determined that the makeup lead to positive changes, including reduction in depression and feelings of inferiority. This is a low-cost and low-risk nonsurgical technique to improve facial reanimation features following nerve injury [27].

5.6.2 Surgical Techniques

There are a plethora of options if surgical correction is chosen (Fig. 5.8). Techniques to improve facial paralysis from nerve injury can be classified as either static or dynamic. Static procedures serve to restore symmetry and limit dysfunctional sequelae but typically do not improve facial movement or tone. Static examples include slings, upper eyelid gold weight, and cosmetic procedures such as brow and/or facelifts to help with the repair. The majority of static procedures are applied to help correct brow deformity. Dynamic procedures aim to restore movement and

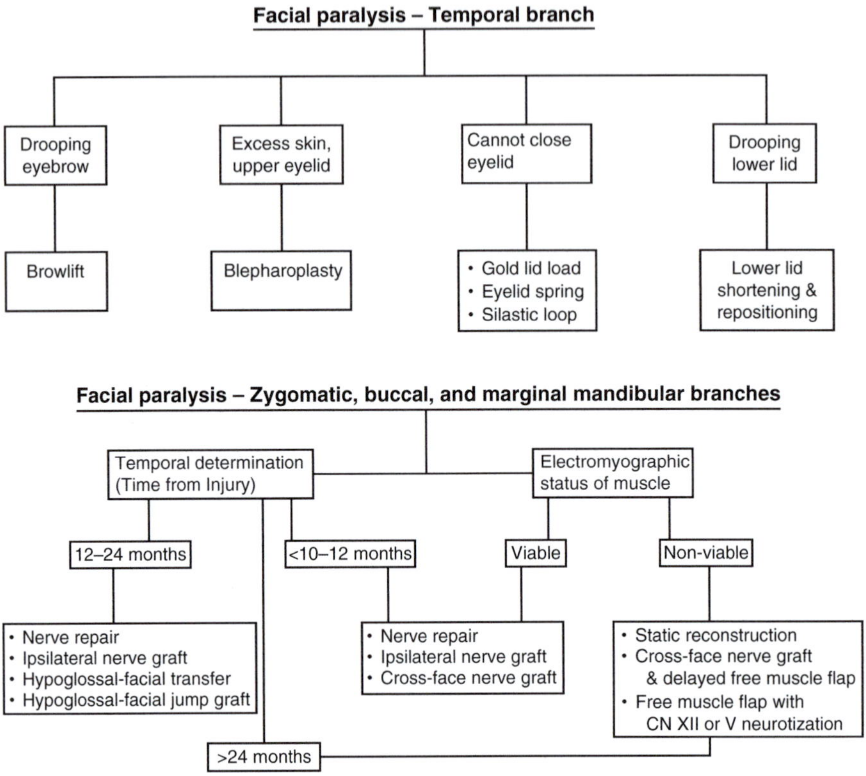

Fig. 5.8 Algorithm for facial nerve injuries with surgical timing and corrective procedures

can be subdivided into neural procedures (cable grafting, cross-facial nerve grafting, and microvascular free flaps) or other procedures such as transposition of the temporalis or masseter and temporalis tendon transfer [15]. Examples of common procedures are described as follows:

1. Gold weight implantation – upper eyelid paralysis
   Facial paralysis in the eye can lead to changes in vision. The implantation of a static weight to load the upper lid and achieve eye closure has been done since 1960. Gold weight implantation in conjunction with a lateral tarsorrhaphy has shown complete eye closure in 83% of patients. Platinum is a new material that may be of greater benefit compared to gold due to the higher density and biocompatibility. Two negative consequences of this technique include undesirable lid closure when in the supine position due to lid loading and gravity as well as the visible bump that is seen on the upper eyelid when it is closed [22, 28–30].
2. Browlift/blepharoplasty
   Brow ptosis can be an unwanted side effect from facial nerve injury. Correction of the ptosis is accomplished with a unilateral or bilateral browlift. Many reconstructive surgeons advocate that symmetry is better accomplished with bilateral

browlifts in the elderly, while unilateral is usually satisfactory in the younger patient. Browlifts may be completed using endoscopic, direct, or mid-forehead approaches [31]. The lift must be conservative due to the tendency of the procedure itself to impede eye closure. Blepharoplasty may be used for excess upper lid skin, but as with the brow lift, it must be conservative.

3. Static facial sling
   This procedure may help with lower facial rehabilitation by restoring only resting symmetry of the cheek and mouth. It is thought to provide inferior functional outcomes in comparison to temporalis transposition (discussed later in the chapter). Autologous tissue, such as fascia lata, has been used as sling material, but can lead to unpredictable stretching. Other materials employed are Gore-Tex® and AHD allograft, AlloDerm™.[1] The sling may assist with oral competence; however, this procedure is commonly utilized to address asymmetry concerns [32–35].
4. Lower eyelid procedures
   The decision to treat or not mainly will depend on lower lid laxity, which is assessed by the snap test. Medial lower lid laxity can cause the inferior punctum to evert from the globe and result in epiphora. Correction is with a medial canthoplasty. For excess lateral lower lid laxity, producing scleral show or ectropion, a horizontal lid-shortening procedure is indicated [15].
5. Neural procedures
   Regardless of cause, primary nerve anastomosis, in the acute setting, is the technique of choice for repair of a completely disrupted facial nerve. The repair should occur as early as possible, with up to 72 h post-injury. Regardless of technique chosen, tension-free repair is essential to prevent scarring and fibrosis [15].
   A. Extratemporal neurorrhaphy
      The optimal timing of primary neurorrhaphy is immediately following injury to permit coaptation of the nerve ends before scarring and retraction begins. The repair may be completed with either a perineural or epineural repair. Direct end-to-end anastomosis of the proximal and distal ends of a transected facial nerve provides the best chance for return of nerve function with either a 9-0 or 10-0 nylon suture [36].
   B. Cross-face grafting
      Although atypical for repair of the nerve, anastomosis of 30–50% of the buccal and zygomatic branches from the unaffected side is used to innervate contralateral paralyzed nerve branches by way of an interposition graft [15]. These healthy nerve branches are sacrificed (theoretically causing minimal deformity on the normal side), with the ultimate goal of restoring symmetry and some mimetic function on the injured side. This potential to gain improvements on the injured side outweighs this minimal negative consequence. Typically this procedure is only chosen if the period of degeneration has been less than 6 months [37–40].

[1] ™Lifecell, Bridgewater, NJ.

C. Cable grafting

Interpositional facial nerve grafting is used when the proximal and distal ends of the nerve cannot be coapted without tension. Techniques have been developed for grafting anywhere along the length of the facial nerve, from the cerebellopontine angle to the parotid gland. In cases in which less than 10 cm of lengths of nerve graft is used, a contralateral greater auricular nerve graft is harvested [15]. Larger lengths will require sural nerve harvesting.

D. Hypoglossal nerve transfer

The transfer of the hypoglossal nerve is a dependable and effective treatment for situations in which the proximal facial nerve is unavailable but the distal nerve remains anatomically intact. Advantages of this procedure include relatively low degree of technical difficulty and relative short time to movement (usually 4–6 months). The major disadvantage includes donor-site morbidity, specifically ipsilateral paralysis of tongue musculature [41–44].

6. Muscle transposition

These procedures are typically used when nerve grafting is not possible due to degradation of distal nerve fibers. Transposition of the temporalis or masseter muscles can provide tone and dynamic reanimation to the lower face. The temporalis muscle transfer requires the movement of the temporalis belly over the zygomatic arch. This can result in significant cosmetic deformity in the temporal and zygomatic region. Using the temporalis tendon transfer technique will avoid this possible deformity. The temporalis tendon is disinserted from its attachment to the coronoid process and transferred to the lateral commissure or melolabial fold. Masseter can be used as well if the surgeon prefers to avoid a large facial incision. However, there is less muscle to use and the vector of force provides less superior angulation to the corner of the mouth [15, 45, 46].

7. Free muscle flaps

Microvascular free flaps utilize free tissue transfer, including soft tissue and corresponding nerve and vascular supply, to rehabilitate the paralyzed face. These flaps have the possibility to allow for emotional animation in addition to better tone. The procedure is typically two staged in which a cross-facial nerve graft is performed approximately 9–12 months prior to the flap. The most common is the gracilis flap [15, 47, 48].

Conclusion

Temporomandibular joint surgeons must have astute surgical principles to avoid facial nerve injury in approaching the joint. Injury to any of the terminal branches can leave the patient with cosmetic, functional, and psychosocial deficiencies. Facial nerve rehabilitation after injury is a challenge. In the majority of situations, full recovery of spontaneous nerve function is unattainable and realistic goals must be set. The timing and etiology of the injury determines the available treatment options. Primary nerve repair, when indicated, is possibly the best option. Multiple reconstructive techniques may be needed to achieve best results. Therefore, understanding the facial nerve anatomy, the prevention of surgical injuries, and quickly recognizing any injury are important for a TMJ surgeon.

References

1. Hall M, Brown R, Leibowitz M. Facial nerve injury during surgery of the temporomandibular joint: a comparison of two dissection techniques. J Oral Maxillofac Surg. 1985;43:20–3.
2. Weinberg S, Kryshtalsky J. Facial nerve function following temporomandibular joint surgery using the preauricular approach. J Oral Maxillofac Surg. 1992;50:1048–51.
3. Ness G. Arthroplasty and discectomy of the temporomandibular joint. Atlas Oral Maxillofac Surg Clin N AM. 2011;19:177–87.
4. Agarwal CA, Mendenhall SD, Foreman KB, et al. The course of the frontal branch of the facial nerve in relation to fascial planes: an anatomic study. Plast Reconstr Surg. 2010;125(2): 532–7.
5. Al-Kayat A, Bramley P. A modified pre-auricular approach to the temporomandibular joint and malar arch. Br J Oral Surg. 1979;17:91–103.
6. Miloro M, Redlinger S, Pennington DM, et al. In situ location of the temporal branch of the facial nerve. J Oral Maxillofac Surg. 2007;65(12):2469.
7. Woltmann M, de Faveri R, Sgrott EA. Anatomosurgical study of the marginal mandibular branch of the facial nerve for submandibular surgical approach. Braz Dent J. 2006;17(1): 71–4.
8. Callander N. Callander surgical anatomy. In: Anson BJ, Maddock WG, editors. Anatomia Quirugical. Barcelona: Salyat Editores; 1956. p. 133.
9. Hall MB, Brown RW, Leibowitz MS. Facial nerve injury during surgery of the temporomandibular joint: a comparison of two dissection techniques. J Oral Maxillofac Surg. 1982;40:699.
10. Westesson PL, Eriksson L, Liedberg J. The risk of damage to facial nerve, superficial temporal vessels, disk and articular surfaces during arthroscopic examination of the temporomandibular joint. Oral Surg. 1986;62:124–7.
11. Holmlund A, Hellsing G. Arthroscopy of the temporomandibular joint: an autopsy study. Int J Oral Surg. 1985;14:169.
12. Diaz RC, Poti SM, Dobie RA. Tests of facial nerve function – otology, neurotology, and skull base surgery – Ch 169. Cummings otolaryngology. 6th ed. Philadelphia: Editor Elsevier; 2015. 2604–2615
13. Politi M, Toro C, Cian R, Costa F, Robiony M. The deep subfascial approach to the temporomandibular joint. J Oral Maxillofac Surg. 2004;62:1097–102.
14. Liu F, Giannakopoulos H, Quinn P, Granquist E. Retrospective study of facial nerve function following temporomandibular joint arthroplasty using the endaural approach. Craniomaxillofac Trauma Reconstr. 2015;8:88–93.
15. Kang T, Vrabec JT, Giddings N, Terris DJ. Facial nerve grading systems (1985-2002): beyond the House-Brackmann Scale. Otol Neurotol. 2002;23:767–72.
16. House J. Facial nerve grading systems. Laryngoscope. 1983;93:1056–69.
17. House JW, Brackmann DE. Facial nerve grading system. Otolaryngol Head Neck Surg. 1985;93:146.
18. Mattox DE. Clinical disorders of the facial nerve – otology, neurotology, and skull base surgery – Ch 170. Cummings otolaryngology. 6th ed. Philadelphia: Editor Elsevier; 2015. p. 2617–30
19. Crumley RL, Armstrong WB, Byrne PJ. Rehabilitation of facial paralysis – Ch 35. Cummings otolaryngology. 4th ed. Philadelphia: Editor Elsevier; 2005. p. 822–52
20. Dressler D, Schonle PW. Botulinum toxin to suppress hyperkinesia after hypoglossal-facial nerve anastomosis. Eur Arch Otorhinolaryngol. 1990;247:391.
21. Barrs DM. Facial nerve trauma: optimal timing for repair. Laryngoscope. 1991;101:835.
22. Ford CN, Bless DM, Lowery JD. Indirect laryngoscopic approach for injection of botulinum toxin in spasmodic dysphonia. Otolaryngol Head Neck Surg. 1990;103:752.
23. Teixeira LJ, Valbuza JS, Prado GF. Physical therapy for Bell's Palsy (idiopathic facial paralysis). Cochrane Database Syst Rev. 2011;12:CD006283
24. Baricich A, et al. Peripheral facial nerve palsy: how effective is rehabilitation. Otol Neurotol. 2012;33:1188.

25. McElhinny ER, Reich I, Burt B, et al. Treatment of pseduoptosis secondary to aberrant regeneration of the facial nerve with botulinum toxin type A. Ophthal Plast Reconstr Surg. 2013;29(3):175–8.
26. Chua CN, et al. Treatment of aberrant facial nerve regeneration with botulinum toxin A. Orbit. 2004;23:213.
27. Kanzaki J, Ohshiro K, Abe T. Effect of corrective make-up training on patients with facial nerve paralysis. Ear Nose Throat J. 1998;77(4):270–4.
28. Freeman MS, et al. Surgical therapy of the eyelids in patients with facial paralysis. Laryngoscope. 1990;100:1086.
29. Jelks GW, Smith B, Bosniak S. The evaluation and management of the eye in facial palsy. Clin Plast Surg. 1979;6:397.
30. Moser G, Oberascher G. Reanimation of the paralyzed face with new gold weight implants and Goretex soft-tissue patches. Eur Arch Otorhinolaryngol. 1997;254(Suppl 1):S76.
31. Moody FP, et al. Endoscopic frontal branch neurectomy, corrugator myectomy, and brow life for forehead asymmetry after facial nerve palsy. Plast Reconstr Surg. 2001;108:218.
32. Anonsen CK, et al. Reinnervation of skeletal muscle with a neuromuscular pedicle. Otolaryngol Head Neck Surg. 1985;93:48.
33. Levine R. Eyelid reanimation surgery. In: May M, editor. The facial nerve. New York: Thieme; 1986.
34. Morel-Fatio D, Lalardrie JP. Palliative surgical treatment of facial paralysis: the palpebral spring. Plast Reconstr Surg. 1964;33:446.
35. McCabe BF. Facial nerve grafting. Plast Reconstr Surg. 1970;45:70–5.
36. Shindo M. Facial reanimation with microneurovascular free flaps. Facial Plast Surg. 2000;16:357.
37. Samii M. Nerves of the head and neck: management of peripheral nerve problems. In: Omer G, Spinner M, editors. Management of peripheral nerve problems. Philadelphia: WB Saunders; 1970.
38. Smith JD, Crumley RL, Harker LA. Facial paralysis in the newborn. Otolaryngol Head Neck Surg. 1981;89:1021.
39. Sachs ME, Conley J. Dual simultaneous systems for facial reanimation. Arch Otolaryngol. 1983;109:137.
40. Ducker TB, Kempe LG, Hayes GJ. The metabolic background for peripheral nerve surgery. J Neurosurg. 1969;30:270.
41. May M, Sobol SM, Mester SJ. Hypoglossal-facial nerve interpositional-jump graft for facial reanimation without tongue atrophy. Otolaryngol Head Neck Surg. 1991;104:818.
42. Arion HG. Dynamic closure of the lids in paralysis of the orbicularis muscle. Int Surg. 1972;57:48.
43. Smith JW. A new technique of facial reanimation. Transactions of fifth international congress of plastic and reconstructive surgery. Chastwood: Butterworths; 1971.
44. Kohs KS, et al. Hypoglossal-facial crossover in facial nerve palsy: pure end-to-side anastomosis technique. Br J Plast Surg. 2002;55:25.
45. Atlas MD, Lowinger DS. A new technique for hypoglossal-facial nerve repair. Laryngoscope. 1997;107:984.
46. Conley J, Miehlke A. Factors influencing results in extratemporal facial nerve repair. In: Fisch U, editor. Facial nerve surgery. Birmingham: Aesculapius Publishing; 1977.
47. Scott AB, Kennedy RA, Stubbs HA. Botulinium A Toxin injection as a treatment for blepharospasm. Arch Ophthalmol. 1985;103:347.
48. Jiang H, et al. One-stage microneurovascular free abductor halluces muscle transplantation for reanimation of facial paralysis. Plast Reconstr Surg. 1995;96:78.

Frey Syndrome

6

Michael D. Chambers and William Chung

6.1 Introduction

Frey syndrome, also known as gustatory sweating or auriculotemporal syndrome, consists of sweating and flushing of the skin in the preauricular area during mastication. Occasionally, a patient may also experience pain in the region. The onset of symptoms is quite variable. Duphenix first described the syndrome in literature in 1757, followed by Baillarger in 1853, and again by Weber in 1897; however, the pathophysiology of the syndrome remained uncertain until 1923 [1–3]. The syndrome itself was named after a Polish neurologist at the University of Warsaw, Lucja Frey, who correctly identified the autonomic innervation of the parotid gland via the auriculotemporal nerve while caring for a patient who sustained a traumatic gunshot wound to the parotid region and exhibited symptoms of gustatory sweating while eating [4].

6.2 Pathophysiology

The auriculotemporal nerve, a branch of the trigeminal nerve, is a mixed nerve that carries general somatosensory fibers as well as parasympathetic and sympathetic fibers. In a normal patient, the parasympathetic fibers stimulate parotid gland salivary secretion, vasodilation, and the erector pilae of the overlying skin. Sympathetic fibers stimulate vasoconstriction of the vessels in the gland, the skin of the preauricular region, and the cutaneous sweat glands. The neurotransmitter released by the parasympathetic nerves at the effector organ is acetylcholine, while that of the sympathetic nerves is norepinephrine.

The pathophysiology of Frey syndrome describes an aberrant process in which the postganglionic parasympathetic nerve fibers innervate the sweat glands and

M.D. Chambers, DMD, MD • W. Chung, DDS, MD (✉)
Oral & Maxillofacial Surgery, University of Pittsburgh Medical Center, Pittsburgh, PA, USA
e-mail: chungwl@upmc.edu

G.F. Bouloux (ed.), *Complications of Temporomandibular Joint Surgery*,
DOI 10.1007/978-3-319-51241-9_6

subcutaneous vascular plexus rather than the secretomotor cells of the parotid gland. This is typically a result of surgery involving the parotid gland such as a parotidectomy or incision and drainage of a parotid abscess. However, there are reports of gustatory sweating associated with blunt trauma to the region, mandibular condyle fractures, temporomandibular joint surgery, and rare congenital abnormalities such as a bifid or trifid condyle [5, 6]. While congenital abnormalities of the condylar head are rare, Blackwood introduced the developmental theory in 1957 which states that a bifid condyle is the result of the fetal vascular fiber septum in the condylar cartilage and its lack of normal involution around 9 weeks of life after birth. The mechanism by which Frey syndrome develops in such a congenital abnormality is unclear [7]. The close anatomical relationship between the auriculotemporal nerve and the temporomandibular joint capsule is of significant importance when operating in the region and results in frequent injury to the nerve with resulting paresthesia and the potential to develop Frey syndrome.

6.3 Frey Syndrome and the Temporomandibular Joint

While Frey syndrome is a frequent outcome following a parotidectomy [8], the risk of developing it with the preauricular approach to the temporomandibular joint is far less. In 1982, Dolwick and Kretzschmar studied the prevalence of various postoperative complications following the surgical treatment of internal derangement of the temporomandibular joint through the preauricular and perimeatal approaches [9]. Fifty-six patients were included in the study with all patients developing paresthesia over the distribution of the auriculotemporal nerve, but no cases of gustatory sweating were reported. A similar study by Kryshtalsky and Weinberg several years later determined that three out of 16 patients demonstrated a positive Minor's starch iodine test after having undergone a similar preauricular approach [10]. Interestingly none of the affected patients admitted to symptomatic gustatory sweating, erythema, or pain in the region.

The previously mentioned studies utilized a preauricular incision that extended inferiorly to the level of the tragus and superiorly in an oblique fashion into the hairline. This larger incision allowed for extensive anterior reflection of the parotid tissues. In 1991, Swanson and Laskin performed a retrospective investigation of 47 temporomandibular joint surgeries using a conservative, straight preauricular incision without the oblique extension and aggressive reflection of the anterior parotid tissues. Twenty-eight patients (47 TMJs) were evaluated with none reporting any subjective gustatory sweating or having a positive Minor's starch iodine test [11]. It remains unclear whether a conservative incision when accessing the temporomandibular joint reduces the likelihood of Frey syndrome.

6.4 Diagnostic Testing

The total hyperhidrotic surface area varies with each Frey syndrome patient (Fig. 6.1). For this reason, it is crucial to accurately map the affected area prior to proceeding with long-term treatment. Minor's iodine starch test, first published in 1927, has remained the traditional method for the evaluation for gustatory sweating [12]. After thoroughly cleaning and drying the area in question, the skin is painted with a layer of 2% iodine solution and allowed to dry. A starch powder is then applied evenly over the site. The patient then chews a piece of gum for several minutes. If Frey syndrome is present, the patient will begin to sweat with the moistened starch reacting with the iodine to produce a dark blue discoloration on the skin surface (Fig. 6.2). The active fraction of the starch is amylose, a polymer

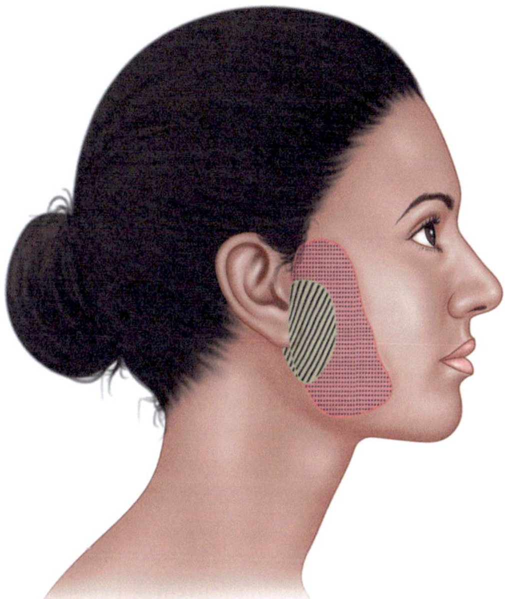

Fig. 6.1 Drawing of positive discoloration with consistent extension (*striped area*) and variable extension (*stippled area*) from Linder et al. [8]

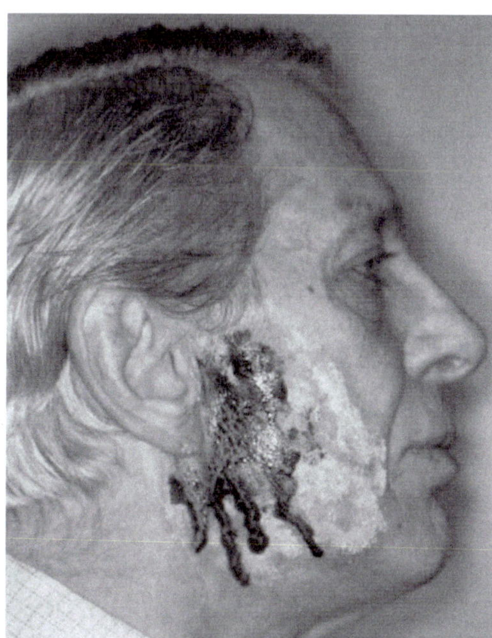

Fig. 6.2 Minor's starch iodide test on a patient with symptomatic gustatory sweating from Linder et al. [8]

of the sugar a-D-glucose, which reacts the small molecules of iodine causing the blue color change [13]. This technique allows the surgeon to determine the precise borders of the affected area in preparation for preventive therapy.

6.5 Treatment

For those patients with symptomatic gustatory sweating, the first line of treatment includes management with antiperspirant deodorants or anticholinergics like scopolamine cream. These treatments only provide temporary relief of symptoms, but may allow patients a functional level of tolerance. For those patients in which conservative treatment is unacceptable, botulinum toxin type A has become the treatment of choice for both long-term control or eradication of the gustatory sweating. Drobik and Laskawi were the first to publish the use of subcutaneous Botox as an effective treatment of gustatory sweating [14]. Botulinum toxin acts by binding presynaptically to high-affinity recognition sites at the cholinergic nerve terminals. Once internalized it binds to SNARE proteins effectively preventing the fusion of synaptic vesicles with the axon membrane. This in turn prevents the release of acetylcholine, causing an overall neuromuscular blocking effect. The Botox is to be delivered at the level of the superficial dermis and usually diffuses within a 5 mm radius. A visible wheal confirms placement in the proper plane of the skin. If the injections are too deep, the muscles of the face may be temporarily weakened, and this risk factor should be openly discussed with the patient prior to treatment. For patients who develop resistance or in which treatment with botulinum toxin type A is ineffective, botulinum toxin type B has been shown to be an effective alternative [15]. The dose of botulinum toxin A needed varies but generally falls between 0.5 and 2.5 units per cm^2.

Occasionally, there are circumstances when Frey syndrome is inadequately treated medically, and therapeutic surgical intervention is necessary. Various flaps have been used prophylactically at the time of parotid resection or postoperatively, after gustatory sweating has developed. These flaps not only act as a physical barrier to prevent abnormal connection between the parasympathetic and sympathetic fibers of the auriculotemporal nerve but also can provide soft tissue bulk to improve a cosmetic deformity after resection of the parotid gland. The sternocleidomastoid, superficial musculoaponeurotic system (SMAS), and temporoparietal fascia flaps have all been reported in literature to decrease or eradicate gustatory sweating [16–18]. In addition to autologous barriers, numerous implants have also been proposed. AlloDerm,™[1] an acellular dermal matrix, is one such implant. It has been shown to reduce the incidence of Frey syndrome effectively and safely and improve overall facial contour [19]. The clinical approach to both physical diagnosis and treatment of gustatory sweating is relatively simple (Fig. 6.3).

[1] ™LifeCell, Bridgewater, NJ, USA.

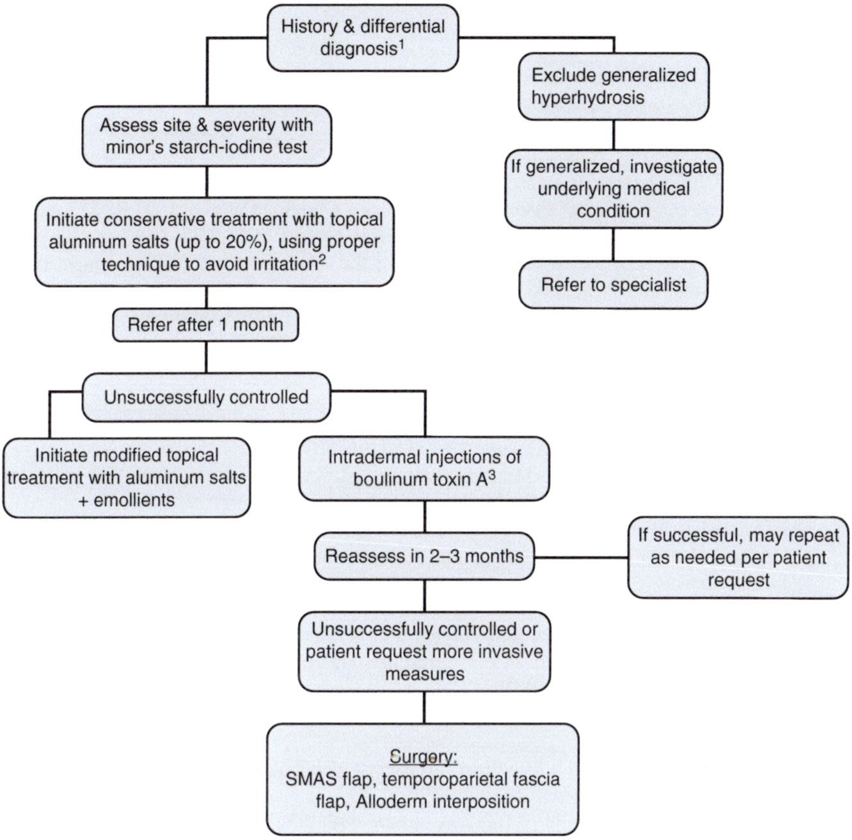

[1] Patients may also request to have no treatment.
[2] Apply to dry area at bedtime, wash off in 6-8hrs. Use 3-7 times/week until euhidrotic. Maintenance treatment every 1-3 wks.
[3] May require nerve block or alternative anesthetic technique because of procedural pain.

Fig. 6.3 Treatment algorithm for Frey syndrome from Clayman et al. [5]

Conclusion

Symptomatic gustatory sweating can have obvious negative social, physical, and psychological implications. Several treatments exist that have proven long-term success in treating Frey syndrome. The prevention of potential complications is a fundamental concept in any surgical treatment plan. The use of a shorter incision in temporomandibular joint surgery may be one avenue for reducing the likelihood of developing Frey syndrome. The reduced surgical access and potential for increased force when retracting while using a shorter incision which may result in facial nerve injury should be carefully considered before choosing this approach.

References

1. Duphenix M. Observations sur les fistules du canal salivaire de Stenon. I Sur une playe compliquee a la joue ou le canal salivaire fut dechire. Mem Acad Royal Chir. 1757;3:431–7.
2. Baillarger M. Mémoire sur l'oblitération du canal de Sténon. Gazette Médicale de Paris. 1853;23:194–7.
3. Weber FP. Clinical cases, V: a case of localized sweating and blushing on eating, possibly due to temporary compression of vasomotor fibers. Trans Clin Soc London. 1897;31:277–80.
4. Frey L. Le syndrome du nerf auriculo-temporal. Rev Neurol. 1923;2:92–104.
5. Clayman M, Clayman S, Seagle M. A review of the surgical and medical treatment of frey syndrome. Ann Plast Surg. 2006;57(5):581–4.
6. Motta-Junior J, Aita G, Pererira-Stabile C, et al. Congenital frey's syndrome associated with nontraumatic bilateral trifid mandibular condyle. Int J Oral Maxillofac Surg. 2013;42:237–9.
7. Blackwood H. The double-headed mandibular condyle. Am J Phys Anthropol. 1957;15(1):1–8.
8. Linder T, Huber A, Schmid S. Frey's syndrome after parotidectomy: a restrospective and prospective analysis. Laryngoscope. 1997;107(11):1496–501.
9. Dolwick M, Kretzschmar D. Morbidity associated with the preauricular and perimeatal approaches to the temporomandibular joint. J Oral Maxillofac Surg. 1982;40:699.
10. Kryshtalskyj B, Weinberg S. An assessment for auriculotemporal syndrome following temporomandibular joint surgery through the preauricular approach. J Oral Maxillofac Surg. 1989;47:3–6.
11. Swanson K, Laskin D, Campbell R. Auriculotemporal syndrome following the preauricular approach to temporomandibular joint surgery. J Oral Maxillofac Surg. 1991;49:680–2.
12. Minor V. Ein neues Verfahren zu der klinischen Untersuchung der Schweissabsonderung. Dtsch Z Nervenheilkd. 1927;101:302–3.
13. Harris D. Quantitative chemical analysis. 7th ed. New York: W.H. Freeman and Company; 2007.
14. Drobik D, Laskawi R. Frey's Syndrome: treatment with botulinum toxin. Acta Otolaryngol. 1995;115(3):459–61.
15. Cantarella G, et al. Treatment of frey's syndrome with botulinum toxin type B. Otolaryngol Head Neck Surg. 2010;143:214–8.
16. Kornblut A, Westphal P, Miehlke A. The effectiveness of a sternocleidomastoid muscle flap in preventing post-parotidectomy occurrence of the Frey syndrome. Acta Otolaryngol. 1974;77:368–73.
17. Casler J, Conley J. Sternocleidomastoid muscle transfer and superficial musculoaponeurotic system plication in the prevention of Frey's syndrome. Laryngoscope. 1991;101:95–100.
18. Cesteleyn L, et al. Temporoparietal fascia flaps and superficial musculoaponeurotic system plication in parotid surgery reduces Frey's syndrome. J Oral Maxillofac Surg. 2002;60:1284–97.
19. Zeng X, et al. AlloDerm implants for prevention of Frey syndrome after parotidectomy: a systematic review and meta-analysis. Mol Med Rep. 2012;5(4):974–80.

Neuropathic Pain and Chronic Opioid Use

7

Ryan Mirchel, John R. Zuniga, and Gary F. Bouloux

7.1 Introduction

Neuropathic pain is defined as pain caused by a lesion of the somatosensory system [1]. The etiologic source located within the somatosensory system differentiates neuropathic pain from nociceptive pain, which by definition represents the processing of noxious stimuli by a functional nervous system [2]. A broad range of disease and injury can result in neuropathic pain and there are multiple classification schema ranging from anatomic to etiologic; none are as of yet universally accepted. Generally, neuropathic pain can be subdivided into four classes:

1. Focal lesions of the peripheral nervous system
2. Generalized lesions of the peripheral nervous system
3. Lesions of the central nervous system
4. Complex neuropathies [3]

Neuropathic pain can be further divided into two broad groups by history and symptoms experienced by the patient: stimulus-evoked and stimulus-independent. Stimulus-evoked pain is characterized by the clinical entities *allodynia*,

R. Mirchel, DDS, MD
Division Oral and Maxillofacial Surgery, Department of Surgery, University of Cincinnati College of Medicine, Cincinnati, OH, USA

J.R. Zuniga, DMD, MS, PhD (✉)
Departments of Surgery and Neurology & Neurotherapeutics, University of Texas Southwestern Medical Center at Dallas, Dallas, TX, USA
e-mail: john.zuniga@utsouthwestern.edu

G.F. Bouloux, MD, DDS, MDSc, FRACDS(OMS), FACS
Division of Oral and Maxillofacial Surgery, Department of Surgery, Emory University School of Medicine, Atlanta, GA, USA
e-mail: gfboulo@emory.edu

G.F. Bouloux (ed.), *Complications of Temporomandibular Joint Surgery*,
DOI 10.1007/978-3-319-51241-9_7

hyperpathia, and *hyperalgesia*. Allodynia is a sensation of pain evoked by a stimulus which would normally not elicit pain. Hyperpathia represents an explosive response to a painful stimulus that temporally outlasts the stimulus on removal. Hyperalgesia is an increased pain response out of proportion to a stimulus which would in normal circumstances cause pain. Stimulus-independent neuropathic pain represents persistent or spontaneous pain unassociated with a causative factor. Stimulus-independent pain is often burning and lancinating and can represent involvement of the sympathetic nervous system [4].

7.2 Pathophysiology

7.2.1 Stimulus-Evoked Pain

Stimulus-evoked pain appears to result in part from central sensitization of the dorsal horn neurons resulting from continuous input from spontaneously firing C-fibers post-injury. This is mediated by N-methyl-D-aspartate (NMDA) receptor sensitization through a biochemical signal cascade involving Substance P and activated protein kinase C [5]. In addition to hyperalgesia, hyperpathia, allodynia, and the universal sensory loss, central sensitization results in a spreading localization of pain from the site of the initial injury [6]. This is commonly noted in the *neuroma*, the swelling found at the proximal end of the injured nerve which contains the regenerative terminal nerve fibers.

In patients who exhibit *only* allodynia, the pathophysiologic process may be related to different processes: A-fiber sprouting and peripheral disinhibition. A-fiber sprouting represents a physiologic response to injury of C-fibers that induces growth of A-fiber terminals in the dorsal horn, which includes the anatomic areas of the dorsal horn where A-fibers are not normally found (Lamina II). These areas are primarily related to pain processing which can induce allodynia. Peripheral disinhibition represents a decreased inhibitory signaling of the dorsal horn neuron by the injured peripheral neuron [7].

7.2.2 Stimulus-Independent Pain

Stimulus-independent pain can be either the more common sodium channel-mediated variety or the less common sympathetically mediated type. After injury to the nerve, accumulation of sodium channels, normally only found in pain-transmitting C-fibers, occurs in the neuroma and along the length of the axon. This results in constitutive hyperexcitability and ectopy, resulting in baseline pain and paresthesia.

Sympathetically mediated neuropathic pain results from a similar process, where after nerve injury axons begin expressing α-adrenoreceptors, sensitizing them to the effects of the sympathetic arm of the nervous system, as well as normally circulating catecholamines [8]. Genetic variation in the catechol-O-methyltransferase (COMT) moiety of the sympathetic nervous system also affects the sensitivity of individuals to pain; 10% of the alleles in the population represent the high pain sensitivity type which corresponds to a low-function enzyme. As an interesting corollary, the incidence of temporomandibular joint disorder (TMD) is significantly lower (2.3-fold) in groups with at least one allele of the high-functioning (low pain sensitivity) COMT gene [9]. While this may indicate the most likely patients to experience TMD also have high pain sensitivities, potentially increasing their risk for neuropathic pain, the theory that COMT polymorphisms affect the evolution of neuropathic pain syndromes is currently equivocal [10, 11].

7.3 Prevention of Neuropathic Pain in Temporomandibular Joint Surgery

A discussion of the prevention of neuropathic pain in temporomandibular joint surgery is made difficult by the paucity of quality evidence surrounding its exact incidence, comorbid, and causative factors. However, we can draw several corollaries from the general evidence on neuropathic and postsurgical pain.

Prevention of neuropathic pain complications should start with the identification of risk factors in the presumptive surgical patient. Genetic polymorphisms in the COMT line can affect sensitivity to pain, and the susceptibility to neuropathic pain has been determined to have a significant genetic component though no specific gene products have been identified [12]. Psychosocial factors such as anxiety, depression, catastrophizing behavior, and perceived social support have also been linked to the postoperative experience of pain. There is a significant correlation between the severity of immediate postoperative pain and the risk of the development of chronic postsurgical pain [13–15], which has led to the development of preoperative pain grading schema in several surgical specialties [16, 17]. It is currently equivocal as to whether or not aggressive pain control or neural blockade in these patients provides any long-term benefit with regard to chronic postsurgical pain [18]. The most likely significant predictor for neuropathic pain after surgery is the presence of preexisting neuropathic pain [19]. Unfortunately, as many of these factors are also correlated with the evolution of temporomandibular joint disease, circumvention of these issues in a surgical patient may be unavoidable.

Other than these factors, based on the epidemiology of neuropathic pain in TMJ surgery, some conclusions can be drawn. Open surgical techniques have been shown to have a significantly higher rate of nerve damage than arthroscopic techniques, so in a susceptible patient, minimally invasive surgery should be considered whenever possible [20, 21]. Nerve injuries in arthroscopy are thought to evolve secondary to extravasation of irrigation solution, so tight control of flow rate intraoperatively may help prevent these complications [22].

7.4 Recognition of Neuropathic Pain in Temporomandibular Joint Surgery

While the incidence of neuropathic pain has been well reported in the literature for other procedures in oral and maxillofacial surgery, few reports of persistent (lasting greater than 6 months) neuropathic pain after temporomandibular joint surgery exist

[23–25]. There is relatively good data on the incidence of neural injury during TMJ surgery, as well as the development of persistent neuropathic pain after direct neural insult. Thirty-five percent of patients who develop a peripheral trigeminal nerve injury will go on to develop a chronic nerve injury [26], and 23–45% of patients who seek care for a persistent peripheral trigeminal nerve injury will go on to develop painful dysesthesia [27, 28].

Shevel reported a single incidence of lower lip paresthesia and two cases of buccal nerve paresthesia lasting longer than 6 months in a series of 46 intraoral condylotomies for TMJ derangement [29]. Multiple large, long-term studies of TMJ arthroscopy have been performed with a 0–3.6% incidence of temporary (less than 6 months) paresthesia to the trigeminal nerve reported [22, 30–35]. The majority of the injuries reported were in the distribution of the auriculotemporal branch [22, 33], although involvement of the lingual [35] and inferior alveolar [34, 35] branches was noted as well. In the largest series to date, 115 temporary and two persistent fifth nerve deficits were noted in 3146 patients [30]. The distribution and characteristics of these injuries remain unclear. The majority of these injuries are thought to be related to neuropraxia secondary to the extravasation of irrigation fluid during the procedure. Direct damage to nerves is thought to be rare due to the surgical anatomy of the arthroscopic lateral approach [36]; however, direct injuries have been reported [22, 34], as well as trigeminal-vagal-mediated bradycardia due to direct manipulation of the auriculotemporal branch [37, 38]. The position of the auriculotemporal nerve is intimate to the condyle, on average being found 10–13 mm inferior to the superior surface of the condyle and 1–2 mm posterior to the neck of the condyle [39]. As a result, it is exceptionally susceptible to compressive neural damage during TMJ procedures and from pathology [40]. Development of auriculotemporal (Frey) syndrome due to this damage is a unique case of neural insult and will be considered in a separate chapter. In open procedures utilizing the preauricular approach, rates of temporary auriculotemporal paresthesia have been reported ranging from 13% to 14% [20, 21].

Chronic dysesthesia secondary to temporomandibular joint surgery is rare with few evidence-based guidelines existing regarding the prognosis. It is the opinion of the authors that the prognosis is poor for complete resolution. Temporomandibular joint surgical patients presenting with a dysesthesia are likely to be multiply-operated patients with all the stigmata of chronic pain: central and peripheral sensitization, muscular hyperalgesia, phenotypic and cortical plasticity, as well as having genetic polymorphisms that predispose them to neuropathic pain. In the authors experience with managing this rare complication, successful management of their pain is very difficult.

7.5 Diagnosis of Neuropathic Pain in Temporomandibular Joint Surgery

The diagnostic approach to the patient with postoperative neuropathic pain should start with a focused history and physical examination. Care should be taken to determine the patients' primary cause of concern (hypoesthesia, anesthesia, pain) as well as the time course and inciting injury. If the patient has pain, it should be discerned whether the pain is spontaneous or provoked and any inciting or mitigating factors. To consider a history of pain as possibly neuropathic, the distribution should be neuroanatomically plausible, as should the inciting history [41].

Physical examination should focus on evidence of nerve injury, atrophy, or potential self-induced trauma. Palpation at the surgical site can give evidence of the etiology of the neuropathy, as well as the pathophysiology if dysesthesia is present. It is important to evaluate and consider other possible causes of chronic postsurgical pain, as persistent pain due to uncorrected pathology can be a significant confounding factor in determining the diagnosis. A minority of patients presenting with persistent pain postsurgically will have a primarily neuropathic etiology [42].

Neurosensory testing should be carried out as well. Multiple schema for neurosensory testing exist and suffer from the difficulty of standardization. Many advanced methodologies are now under use as well [43]. The authors utilize the three-level dropout clinical neurosensory test developed by Zuniga and Essick [44]. The presence of the defining characteristic of neuropathy should be present in the relevant neuroanatomic distribution [41]. Confirmatory testing should be performed if possible [41], with magnetic resonance neurography offering the best opportunity to locate the precise site of injury [45]. (Fig. 7.1, Tables 7.1 and 7.2)

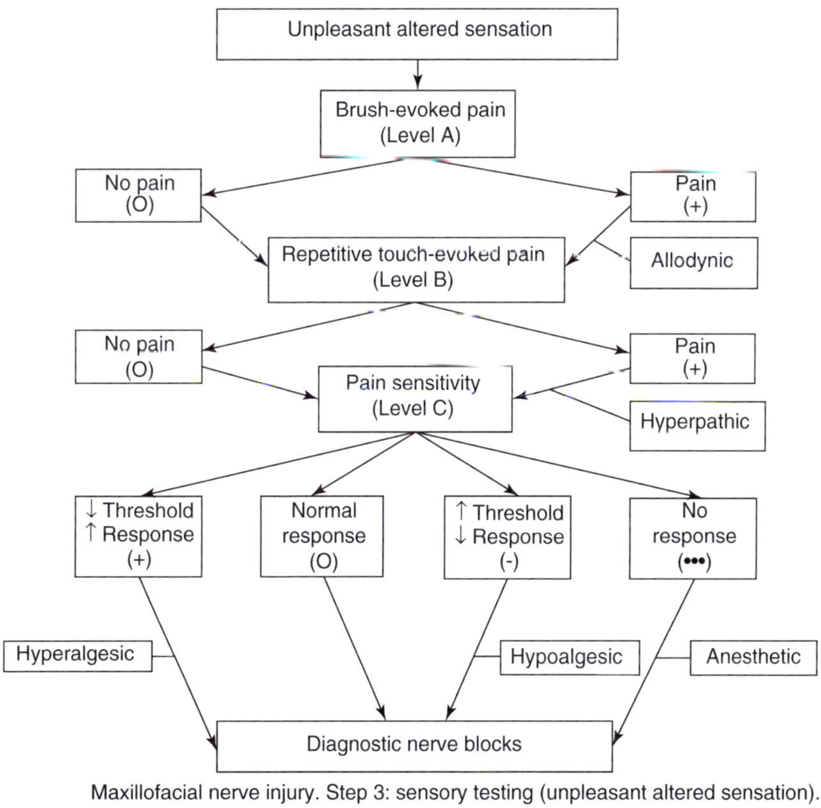

Fig. 7.1 Sensory testing (unpleasant altered sensation) (Adapted from: Zuniga and Essick [44])

Table 7.1 Sensory testing for the patient with unpleasant altered sensation

Level A testing: Test for brush-evoked pain
Normal response—patient does not experience pain in response to brush strokes (*go to level B testing*)
Allodynic patient—experiences pain in response to brush strokes (*go to level B testing*)
Level B testing: Test for repetitive touch-evoked pain
Normal response—patient does not experience pain in response to repetitive application of touch/pressure stimulus (*go to level C testing*)
Hyperpathic patient—experiences pain in response to repetitive application of touch/pressure stimulus (*go to level C testing*)
Level C testing: Pain sensitivity
Normal response—patient exhibits unremarkable response to pin prick, increased pressure (algometer) pain threshold, or increased thermal pain threshold on test site
Hyperalgesia patient—exhibits exaggerated response to pin prick, decreased pressure (algometer) pain threshold, or decreased thermal pain threshold on test site
Hypoalgesia patient—exhibits little response to pin prick, increased pressure (algometer) pain threshold, or increased thermal pain threshold on test site
Anesthetic patient— exhibits no response to pin prick, noxious pressures, and heat on test site

Adapted from: Zuniga and Essick [44]

Table 7.2 Diagnostic criteria for posttraumatic pain dysesthesias neuropathic pain (Jensen et al. [1])

	Spontaneity of pain[a]		Step 3 results[b]			Nerve block results[c]	
Pain disorder	Constant	Intermittent	Level A	Level B	Level C	Peripheral[d]	Stellate ganglion
Neuroma pain	V	T	O	O	or… –	+	
Allodynia	R	R	+	O	O	or… –	
Hyperalgesia	R	R	O	O	+	+	
Hyperpathia	V	T	+	+	oor⁻or⁺	–	–
Sympathetically mediated pain	T	V	+	+	+	–	+
Central trigeminal pathoses	T	V	O	oor⁻	or... –	–	
Anesthesia dolorosa	T	R	O	O	…	–	
Psychogenic pain	V	V	O	O	O		

Adapted from: Zuniga and Essick [43]

[a]*T* typical, *V* variable, *R* rare (information obtained during Step 1)

[b]See Fig. 4 for explanation of symbols

[c]+, pain relieved by block; –, pain not relieved by block; blank, block not usually performed

[d]Proximal to site of injury

7.6 Management of Neuropathic Pain

The management of neuropathic pain secondary to TMJ surgery is likely to be challenging due to the poor prognosis. Appropriate diagnosis of the primary etiology and potential comorbid diseases is essential. Due to the poor prognosis, medical and adjunctive therapy should be the first line of treatment.

There are few high-quality studies specifically addressing the medical treatment of postsurgical peripheral dysesthesia; however, there is excellent data on the medical treatment of neuropathic pain in general. While it is currently unknown to what extent a study evaluating treatment in one neuropathic pain syndrome applies to another unstudied condition, a pattern of effective first-line medications has emerged. Additionally, because of the unpredictable individual variation in treatment response that emerges in the management of chronic neuropathic pain, many patients will require multiple trials of first-line medications regardless. Presented are the most recent International Association for the Study of Pain (IASP) recommendations for the treatment of neuropathic pain [46] and the 2010 update [47] (Tables 7.3 and 7.4).

Table 7.3 Stepwise pharmacologic management of neuropathic pain

Stepwise pharmacologic management of neuropathic pain (NP)
Step 1
Assess pain and establish the diagnosis of NP [20, 25]; if uncertain about the diagnosis, refer to a pain specialist or neurologist
Establish and treat the cause of NP; if uncertain about availability of treatments addressing NP etiology, refer to appropriate specialist
Identify relevant comorbidities (e.g., cardiac, renal, or hepatic disease, depression, gait instability) that might be relieved or exacerbated by NP treatment or that might require dosage adjustment or additional monitoring of therapy
Explain the diagnosis and treatment plan to the patient and establish realistic expectations
Step 2
Initiate therapy of the disease causing NP, if applicable
Initiate symptom treatment with one or more of the following:
A secondary amine TCA (nortriptyline, desipramine) or an SSNRI (duloxetine, venlafaxine)
A calcium channel α2-δ ligand, either gabapentin or pregabalin
For patients with localized peripheral NP, topical lidocaine used alone or in combination with one of the other first-line therapies
For patient with acute neuropathic cancer pain, or episode exacerbations of severe pain, and when prompt pain relief during titration of a first-line medication to an efficacious dosage is required; opioid analgesics or tramadol may be used alone or in combination with one of the first-line therapies
Evaluate patient for non-pharmacologic treatments and initiate if appropriate
Step 3
Reassess pain and health-related quality of life frequently
If substantial pain relief (e.g., average pain reduced to ≤3/10) and tolerable side effects, continue treatment

(continued)

Table 7.3 (continued)

If partial pain relief (e.g., average pain remains ≥4/10) after an adequate trial (see Table 7.3), add one of the other first-line medications
If no or inadequate pain relief (e.g., <30% reduction) at target dosage after an adequate trial (see Table 7.3), switch to an alternative first-line medication
Step 4
If trials of first-line medications alone and in combination fail, consider second- and third-line medications or referral to a pain specialist or multidisciplinary pain center

Adapted from Dworkin et al. [46]
TCA tricyclic antidepressant, *SSNRI* selective serotonin and norepinephrine reuptake inhibitor

Table 7.4 Stepwise pharmacologic management of neuropathic pain [48]

Step 1
Assess pain and establish the diagnosis of NP; if uncertain about the diagnosis, refer to a pain specialist or neurologist
Establish and treat the cause of NP; if uncertain about availability of treatments for cause of NP, refer to appropriate specialist
Identify relevant comorbidities (eg, cardiac, renal, or hepatic disease, depression, gait instability) that might be relieved or exacerbated by NP treatment or that might require dosage adjustment or additional monitoring of therapy
Explain the diagnosis and treatment plan to the patient and establish realistic expectations
Step 2
Initiate therapy for the disease causing NP, if applicable
Initiate symptom treatment with one or more of the following:
A secondary amine TCA (nortriptyline, desipramine) or an SSNRI (duloxetine, venlafaxine)
A calcium channel α_2-δ ligand, either gabapentin or pregabalin
For patients with localized peripheral NP, topical lidocaine used alone or in combination with one of the other first-line therapies
For patients with acute NP, neuropathic cancer pain, or episodic exacerbations of severe pain and when prompt pain relief during titration of a first-line medication to an efficacious dosage is required, opioid analgesics or tramadol may be used alone or in combination with 1 of the first-line therapies
Evaluate patient for nonpharmacological treatments and initiate if appropriate
Step 3
Reassess pain and health-related quality of life frequently
If substantial pain relief (e.g., average pain reduced to ≤3/10) and tolerable adverse effects, continue treatment
If partial pain relief (e.g., average pain remains ≥4/10 after an adequate trial, add one of the other four first-line medications)
If no or inadequate pain relief (e.g., <30% reduction) at target dosage after an adequate trial, switch to an alternative first-line medication
Step 4
If trials of first-line medications alone and in combination fail, consider second- and third-line medications or referral to a pain specialist or multidisciplinary pain center

Adapted from Dworkin et al. [47]
NP neuropathic pain, *SSNRI* selective serotonin norepinephrine reuptake inhibitor, *TCA* tricyclic antidepressant

Additionally, it is worthwhile to consider alternative therapies in these patients, such as cognitive behavioral therapy and sensory retraining [48, 49].

7.7 Chronic Opioid Use

The development of pain within the heterogenous TMD population is generally considered to be multifactorial. This caveat probably also applies, albeit to a lesser extent, to patients with true temporomandibular joint (TMJ) pathology and pain. Most patients with TMJ pathology and pain will respond to nonsurgical treatment although a minority may benefit from surgical intervention. Those patients who undergo surgery typically are managed with a variety of analgesic medications in the postoperative period. The most common medications used include nonsteroidal anti-inflammatory medication, opioids, and adjunct neuromodulating medications such as carbamazepine, gabapentin, pregabalin, lamotrigine, tricyclic antidepressants, and selective serotonin norepinephrine reuptake inhibitors. Postsurgical patient requirements for pain medication may vary from a few days to several weeks depending on many factors including the nature of the surgical procedure; the level of presurgical pain; the duration of the pain symptoms; the number of prior surgical procedures, psychosocial factors, and genetic polymorphisms; and the presence of neuropathic pain (Fig. 7.2).

There are two potential complications that can arise from temporomandibular joint surgery as it relates to pain. The first is the development of a chronic pain state.

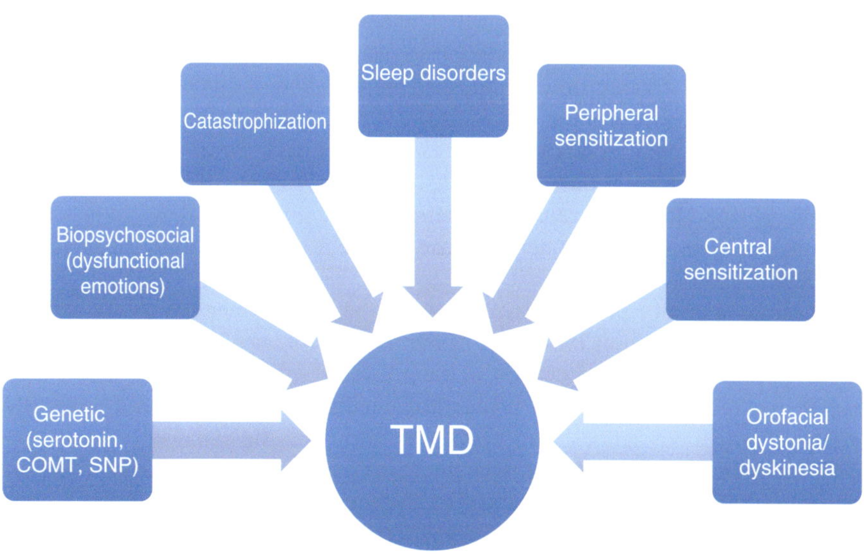

Fig. 7.2 Multifactorial nature of TMD pain

This may be due to the development of pain through peripheral sensitization and/or central sensitization, the failure to recognize the presence of psychosocial issues, the potential for catastrophization or the development of neuropathic pain. It is critical to appreciate and understand the nature of the pain to ensure that additional TMJ surgery is avoided in a feeble attempt to address the pain. The inability to adequately address the chronic pain with NSAIDs, acetaminophen, neuromodulating drugs, and physical therapy may necessitate the use of opioids ranging from weak to strong. This may occasionally result in the long-term use of and dependence on opioids.

The second complication relates to the potential development of adverse drug-related behavior (ADRB) from opioid medications. Opioid misuse remains a major epidemic resulting in significant morbidity and mortality. Opioid misuse is often manifest by patients seeking multiple provider prescriptions, unsanctioned dose escalation, prescription losses, requesting specific opioids, and deteriorating social functioning.

7.7.1 Opioid Tolerance

Most patients will develop tolerance to opioids overtime. The result will typically be the development of increased pain and the requirement for increasing doses of opioids. These events should not signal the development of ADRB. Tolerance can generally be divided into innate and acquired. The former is typically the result of pharmacokinetics and the wide variation in the functionality of the CYP2D6 enzyme which is largely responsible for converting most opioid prodrugs to active compounds. Bhushnan provides an excellent review of pharmacogenetics and chronic pain management [50]. In general, patients may be classified as slow, intermediate, rapid, or ultrarapid metabolizers depending on the nature of the CYP2D6 enzyme. Patients who are slow or intermediate metabolizers would be expected to have lower plasma concentrations of active drugs and less analgesic effect. The methods of developing tolerance differ to some degree between different opioids drugs but the net result is the same. There are also more than 100 single nucleotide polymorphisms (SNP) that result in variations in the μ-receptor affinity for opioids and analgesic response. The net response can be a two- to tenfold difference in analgesic effect.

Pharmacokinetics plays a crucial role in the development of tolerance as a result of the induction or inhibition of metabolic enzymes like CYP2D6 resulting in a time-dependent alteration in the plasma level of active drug. This may result in a reduced fraction of μ-receptor occupation and a reduced analgesic effect. Pharmacodynamics also plays a role in that the intrinsic response to μ-receptor binding by opioids may decrease overtime as a result of receptor phosphorylation and internalization or G-receptor uncoupling. There is also evidence that the primary opioid transporter P-glycoprotein (P-g) which is coded for by the mDR1 gene is responsible to opioid efflux from cells and can be up-regulated in the presence of chronic opioid exposure to increase tolerance.

7.7.2 Pain Ladder

The concept of using a pain ladder originated from World Health Organization guidelines for patients with chronic cancer pain [51]. It provides a simple algorithm to limit the prescription of opioids until the use of all alternative analgesics has been exhausted. A stepwise approach beginning with NSAIDs followed by the use of weak, moderate, and finally strong opioids is generally recommended. The use of adjunct medications is further encouraged as they can be associated with a significant reduction in pain with the number needed to treat (NNT) for a 50% reduction in pain ranging from 3 to 10 [52].

7.7.3 Is There an Opioid Benefit?

Opioids have been shown to achieve a meaningful reduction in pain (30% or greater) in approximately 50% of patients in chronic non-cancer pain for up to 12 weeks [53]. Many patients ultimately discontinue medication as a result of inadequate pain relief or side effects. There is no evidence to support or refute the use of opioids in temporomandibular joint pain and guidelines only reflect expert opinion. Equally important is the goal of improving activities of daily living and quality of life with opioids although there is no evidence to support the use of opioids to improve these outcomes. The limited evidence supporting opioids in the non-cancer chronic pain should not be a reason to withhold them from patients with TMJ pain who may benefit although further studies are clearly needed to clarify the exact role of opioids. Many clinicians choose to prescribe short-acting opioids based in part on a lack of experience with long-acting agents. Short-acting opioids do provide the ability to better control pain that fluctuates throughout the day despite the need for more frequent dosing, issues with patient compliance, and increased risk for ADRB. However, long-acting opioids provide better plasma levels, improved compliance, and reduced ADRB, particularly with abuse-deterrent formulations [54].

The use of opioids to improve function and quality of life in chronic non-cancer pain is less clear [54, 55]. There is some evidence that failure to return to work correlates with opioids in a dose-dependent manner. Functional improvements appear to be better with NSAIDs and weak opioids such as tramadol.

The use of long-term opioids in patients with chronic TMJ pain remains controversial as it does in most chronic non-cancer pain states. A lack of evidence to support chronic opioids should not serve as a reason to withhold them although any long-term prescribing beyond 4 weeks should be weighed carefully balancing the patient analgesic requirement and the potential for ADRB and opioid misuse.

7.7.4 Opioid-Related Adverse Events

Adverse events (AE) include dry mouth, constipation, sweating, weight gain, somnolence, sleep disturbance, memory impairment, fatigue, dizziness, sexual dysfunction, nausea, and urinary retention. The vast majority of patients on opioids will experience at least one AE with the relative risk of any AE being 1.55 [56].

A relatively significant number of patients will ultimately discontinue opioids as a result of AE. This approaches 23% with oral medications and 12% with transdermal medications. Additionally, the lack of adequate pain reduction will lead another 10% and 6% of patients on oral and transdermal medications, respectively, to discontinue treatment [53].

Opioids may result in AE even if there is no ADRB. The most feared AE is respiratory depression as this may be life threatening. This may be the result of drug interactions, particularly with respect to cytochrome P450 enzymes within the liver, or the synergistic effect of additional respiratory depressants such as benzodiazepines and alcohol. The net result is both central and obstructive sleep apnea. The risk of respiratory depression appears to be least when the total daily dose of pain medication is less than an oral morphine equivalent dose of 50 mg.

Drug interactions may also result in serotonin syndrome in patients taking monoamine oxidase inhibitors or antidepressants. The risk appears greatest with meperidine, tramadol, and methadone as these opioids also inhibit serotonin reuptake. Cardiac dysrhythmias are generally unrelated to opioid use unless secondary to respiratory depression. One exception is methadone which can result in a prolonged QTc in some patients and therefore requires close monitoring with electrocardiograms.

Cytochrome P450 enzymes such as CYP2D6 play a crucial role in the metabolism of many drugs including opioids. Polymorphisms within this and additional enzymes ensure that there is a large individual variation between patients. Patients can be classified as ultra-rapid, rapid, intermediate, and poor metabolizers. The former may be associated with opioid toxicity. The challenge lies in identifying those patients at risk.

Opioids also have the potential to cause tolerance, opioid-induced hyperalgesia, immunosuppression, and hypogonadism. Immunosuppression is the result of a decrease in angiogenesis, macrophage, and neutrophil sequestration and natural killer cells. A subset of patients with human immunodeficiency virus may also have disease progression due to the opioid up-regulated expression of the HIV CCR5. Hypogonadism is the result of a reduction in gonadotropin-releasing hormone, luteinizing hormone, follicle-stimulating hormone, and adrenocorticotropic hormone.

7.7.5 Adverse Drug-Related Behavior

Opioid abuse, misuse, and addiction are concerns in any patient receiving opioids. Abuse generally refers to the use of medication to achieve euphoria. Misuse refers to the use of medication in a manner different from that prescribed or continued use despite AE or harm. Addiction refers to the use of medication as a result of "craving" despite harm and complications. The overall risk of ADRB appears to be approximately 20%. The incidence of misuse and addiction is increasing with current figures estimating misuse at 21–29% and addiction at 8–12% [57]. The greatest risk factors appear to be a history of substance abuse, psychiatric diagnoses, and a lack of social support. Many consider that the relatively high rates for ADRB may be the result of "adverse patient selection." The opioid risk tool (ORT) can be used to help predict the likelihood of ADRB although the predictive value remains only modest for moderate to severe ADRB. This tool stratifies patients as low, moderate, or high risk for misuse of opioids. Other questionnaires including the Revised Screener and Opioid Assessment for Patients in Pain (SOAPP) can also be used to assist risk-stratifying patients. Opioid-naïve patients, such as those who are not receiving narcotics but will undergo surgery and require postoperative opioids, have a relative risk (RR) for ADRB of 2.5 and 14.3 if a positive result is identified from the revised SOAPP and the ORT, respectively. These tests are patient administered and need to be completed prior to initiation of opioid medication. Patients who are already receiving opioids can be evaluated for ADRB by using the Current Opioid Misuse Measure (COMM) which is a clinician-administered test with a RR of 2.7 for ADRB with a positive test result [58].

The importance of monthly follow-up visits with the clinician is critical to evaluate pain levels and the response to all pain medications as well as document AE and any suspected ADRB. The role of random urinary drug screening (UDS) to determine both the appropriate presence of opioid and the absence of all non-clinician-sanctioned drugs is generally accepted as reasonable for long-term pain management but may not be beneficial in managing postsurgical patients. Patients who continue to require opioids beyond 3 months may however benefit from UDS in the same way other than chronic pain patients do [59]. The use of random plasma drug screening is more controversial although it provides a unique opportunity to quantitate the plasma level of the prescribed opioid which can be correlated with drug metabolism and the patient response to determine the most ideal dosing and opioid [60]. Patients deemed to be high risk should be managed by dedicated pain specialists.

The single most concerning ADRB is overdose. There are approximately 16,000 opioid-related deaths per year in the USA [61]. An additional 1000 patients per day are seen in emergency departments in the USA for prescription opioid overdoses. The problem is likely to grow as the number of opioid prescriptions increases every year despite increasing awareness and tight regulatory control by the Food and Drug Administration (FDA). The importance of assessing every patient individually and ensuring that psychosocial factors are considered cannot be understated.

The relative risk (RR) for mortality for short- and long-term opioid use is 1.36 and 1.72, respectively. Interestingly the RR for chronic pain patients treated with non-opioid analgesics is 1.39. This would suggest that the mere presence of chronic pain is a risk factor for all-cause mortality with additional risks associated with long-term opioid use [62]. Indeed polypharmacy with NSAIDs and acetaminophen in addition to opioids in an attempt to reduce opioid use is itself associated with increased patient harm [63].

7.7.6 Recommendations

Any patient who will receive an extended period of opioids should have a complete history and physical examination. The history is also very important to help identify patients with psychological issues including anxiety, depression, somatization,

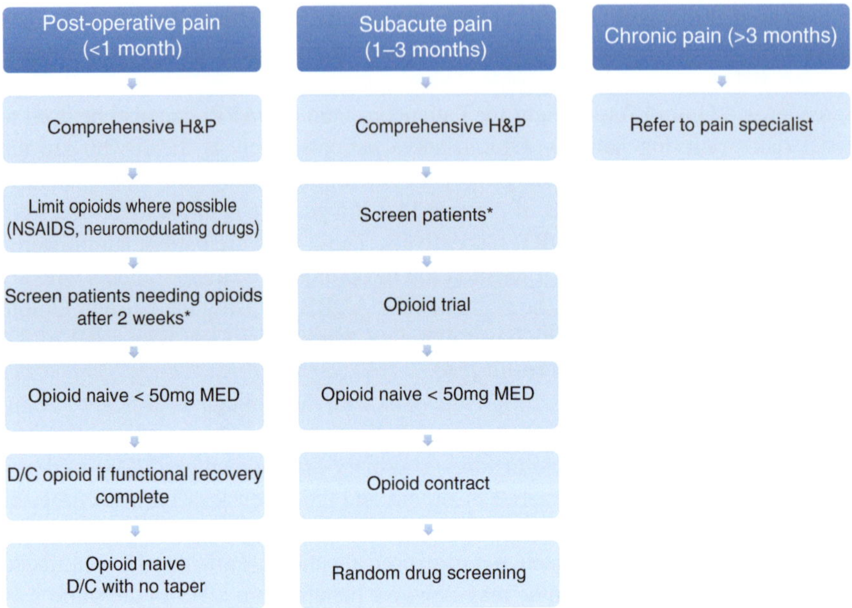

Fig. 7.3 Algorithm for postoperative opioids (Adapted from Hegmann et al. [65])

prior prescription abuse, and other personality traits that would make them both a poor surgical candidate and a poor candidate for opioids. Prior to prescribing opioids, consideration should be given to checking opioid monitoring programs to ensure that other physicians are not also prescribing opioids [64]. The physician should also evaluate the potential for drug/drug and drug/disease interactions as well as consider a written contract to outline the patient and physician responsibilities, obligations, and grounds for termination [59]. Recommendations for the use of perioperative opioids have been developed and serve as a useful guide for physicians [65] (Fig. 7.3).

If long-term opioids are needed, transitioning from immediate release medications to sustained release medications can be achieved by simply replacing the total daily dose of IR medication with the same dose of ER medication if the patient has adequate pain relief. Patients without adequate pain relief can also be transitioned to ER medications using the same method, but progressive dose escalation will be required to achieve adequate pain relief.

Monthly visits should document pain relief, functional activity, side effects, and quality of life. Adverse drug-related behavior should be actively sought. These include prescription forgery, losing prescriptions, dose escalations, requesting specific drugs, and aggressive behavior.

In order to reduce the risks of AE and ADRB, the total daily dose of opioid should ideally be less than 50 mg morphine equivalent dose (MED) which translates to no more than four tablets of oxycodone 10 mg or five tablets of hydrocodone 10 mg per day. Total treatment time should strive for 4 weeks or less and no taper is generally required when the MED is less than 50 mg. Daily doses of opioid in excess of the 50 MED should be discontinued with a 7-day taper to reduce the likelihood of withdrawal.

When it is anticipated that opioids will be needed for more than 4 weeks, it is generally considered appropriate to have a pain contract that clearly outlines the physician and patient responsibilities as well as the consequences of violating the agreement. The use of UDS should also be considered to monitor for compliance, a lack of diversion, and the ingestion of other nonphysician-endorsed drugs. This should be performed at least every 3 months for daily doses less than 50 mg MED and monthly for daily doses greater than 50 mg MED.

References

1. Jensen TS, Baron R, Haanpää M, et al. A new definition of neuropathic pain. Pain. 2011;152:2204–5.
2. Gilron I, Jensen TS, Dickenson AH. Combination pharmacotherapy for management of chronic pain: from bench to bedside. Lancet Neurol. 2013;12:1084–95.
3. Freynhagen R, Bennett MI. Diagnosis and management of neuropathic pain. BMJ. 2009;339:b3002.
4. Woolf CJ, Mannion RJ. Neuropathic pain: etiology, symptoms, mechanisms, and management. Lancet. 1999;353(9168):1959–64.
5. Chen L, Huang LY. Protein kinase C reduces Mg2+ block of NMDA-receptor channels as a mechanism of modulation. Nature. 1992;356(6369):521–3.
6. Koelbaek Johansen M, Graven-Nielsen T, Schou Olesen A, Arendt-Nielsen L. Generalized muscular hyperalgesia in chronic whiplash syndrome. Pain. 1999;83(2):229–34.
7. Woolf CJ, Shortland P, Coggeshall RE. Peripheral nerve injury triggers central sprouting of myelinated afferents. Nature. 1992;355(6355):75–8.
8. McMahon SB, Koltzenburg M, Tracey I, et al. Wall & Melzack's textbook of pain, expert consult – Online and Print. In: Wall & Melzack's textbook of pain. 6th ed. Philadelphia: Elsevier Health Sciences; 2013.
9. Diatchenko L, Slade GD, Nackley AG, et al. Genetic basis for individual variations in pain perception and the development of a chronic pain condition. Hum Mol Genet. 2005;14(1):135–43.
10. Armero P, Muriel C, Santos J, Sànchez-Montero FJ, Rodrógeuz RE, González-Sarmiento R. COMT (Val158Met) polymorphism is not associated to neuropathic pain in a Spanish population. Eur J Pain. 2005;9(3):229–32.
11. Calcutt NA. Potential mechanisms of neuropathic pain in diabetes. Int Rev Neurobiol. 2002;50:205–28.
12. Devor M, Raber P. Heritability of symptoms in an experimental model of neuropathic pain. Pain. 1990;42(1):51–67.
13. Caumo W, Schmidt AP, Schneider CN, et al. Preoperative predictors of moderate to intense acute postoperative pain in patients undergoing abdominal surgery. Acta Anaesthesiol Scand. 2002;46(10):1265–71.
14. Hanley MA, Jensen MP, Ehde DM, Hoffman AJ, Patterson DR, Robinson LR. Psychosocial predictors of long-term adjustment to lower-limb amputation and phantom limb pain. Disabil Rehabil. 2004;26(14–15):882–93.
15. Perkins FM, Kehlet H. Chronic pain as an outcome of surgery. A review of predictive factors. Anesthesiology. 2000;93(4):1123–33.
16. Werner MU, Duun P, Kehlet H. Prediction of postoperative pain by preoperative nociceptive responses to heat stimulation. Anesthesiology. 2004;100(1):115–9.

17. Granot M, Lowenstein L, Yarnitsky D, Tamir A, Zimmer EZ. Post cesarean section pain prediction by preoperative experimental pain assessment. Anesthesiology. 2003;98(6):1422–6.
18. Ong CK, Lirk P, Seymour RA, Jenkins BJ. The efficacy of preemptive analgesia for acute postoperative pain management: a meta-analysis. Anesth Analg. 2005;100(3):757–73, table of contents.
19. Zuniga JR, Yates DM, Phillips CL. The presence of neuropathic pain predicts postoperative neuropathic pain following trigeminal nerve repair. J Oral Maxillofac Surg. 2014;72(12): 2422–7.
20. Smith JA, Sandler NA, Ozaki WH, Braun TW. Subjective and objective assessment of the temporalis myofascial flap in previously operated temporomandibular joints. J Oral Maxillofac Surg. 1999;57(9):1058–65.
21. Dolwick MF, Kretzschmar DP. Morbidity associated with the preauricular and perimeatal approaches to the temporomandibular joint. J Oral Maxillofac Surg. 1982;40(11):699–700.
22. González-garcía R, Rodríguez-campo FJ, Escorial-hernández V, et al. Complications of temporomandibular joint arthroscopy: a retrospective analytic study of 670 arthroscopic procedures. J Oral Maxillofac Surg. 2006;64(11):1587–91.
23. Kipp DP, Goldstein BH, Weiss WW. Dysesthesia after mandibular third molar surgery: a retrospective study and analysis of 1,377 surgical procedures. J Am Dent Assoc. 1980;100(2):185–92.
24. Politis C, Lambrichts I, Agbaje JO. Neuropathic pain after orthognathic surgery. Oral Surg Oral Med Oral Pathol Oral Radiol. 2014;117(2):e102–7.
25. Renton T, Yilmaz Z. Profiling of patients presenting with posttraumatic neuropathy of the trigeminal nerve. J Orofac Pain. 2011;25(4):333–44.
26. Kipp DP, Goldstein BH, Weiss WW. Dysesthesia after mandibular third molar surgery: a retrospective study and analysis of 1,377 surgical procedures. J Am Dent Assoc. 1980;100(2):185–92.
27. Jääskeläinen SK, Teerijoki-oksa T, Forssell H. Neurophysiologic and quantitative sensory testing in the diagnosis of trigeminal neuropathy and neuropathic pain. Pain. 2005;117(3): 349–57.
28. Pogrel MA, et al. Long-term outcome of trigeminal nerve injuries related to dental treatment. J Oral Maxillofac Surg. 2011;69(9):2284–8.
29. Shevel E. Intra-oral condylotomy for the treatment of temporomandibular joint derangement. Int J Oral Maxillofac Surg. 1991;20(6):360–1.
30. McCain JP, Sanders B, Koslin MG, et al. Temporomandibular joint arthroscopy: a 6-year multicenter retrospective study of 4,831 joints. J Oral Maxillofac Surg. 1992;50(9):926–30.
31. Zhang S, Yang C, Cai X, et al. Prevention and treatment for the rare complications of arthroscopic surgery in the temporomandibular joint. J Oral Maxillofac Surg. 2011;69(11): e347–53.
32. Silva PA, Lopes MT, Freire FS. A prospective study of 138 arthroscopies of the temporomandibular joint. Braz J Otorhinolaryngol. 2015;81(4):352–7.
33. Tsuyama M, Kondoh T, Seto K, Fukuda J. Complications of temporomandibular joint arthroscopy: a retrospective analysis of 301 lysis and lavage procedures performed using the triangulation technique. J Oral Maxillofac Surg. 2000;58(5):500–5.
34. Heffez L, Blaustein D. Diagnostic arthroscopy of the temporomandibular joint. Part I: normal arthroscopic findings. Oral Surg Oral Med Oral Pathol. 1987;64(6):653–70.
35. Carls FR, Engelke W, Locher MC, Sailer HF. Complications following arthroscopy of the temporomandibular joint: analysis covering a 10-year period (451 arthroscopies). J Craniomaxillofac Surg. 1996;24(1):12–5.
36. Westesson PL, Eriksson L, Liedberg J. The risk of damage to facial nerve, superficial temporal vessels, disk, and articular surfaces during arthroscopic examination of the temporomandibular joint. Oral Surg Oral Med Oral Pathol. 1986;62(2):124–7.
37. Gomez TM, Van Gilder JW. Reflex bradycardia during TMJ arthroscopy: case report. J Oral Maxillofac Surg. 1991;49(5):543–4.

38. Roberts RS, Best JA, Shapiro RD. Trigeminocardiac reflex during temporomandibular joint arthroscopy: report of a case. J Oral Maxillofac Surg. 1999;57(7):854–6.
39. Fernandes PR, De Vasconsellos HA, Okeson JP, Bastos RL, Maia ML. The anatomical relationship between the position of the auriculotemporal nerve and mandibular condyle. Cranio. 2003;21(3):165–71.
40. Ansari H, Robertson CE, Lane JI, Viozzi CF, Garza I. Auriculotemporal neuralgia secondary to TMJ synovial cyst: a rare presentation of a rare entity. Headache. 2013;53(10):1662–5.
41. Treede RD, Jensen TS, Campbell JN, et al. Neuropathic pain: redefinition and a grading system for clinical and research purposes. Neurology. 2008;70(18):1630–5.
42. Dualé C, Ouchchane L, Schoeffler P, Dubray C. Neuropathic aspects of persistent postsurgical pain: a French multicenter survey with a 6-month prospective follow-up. J Pain. 2014;15(1):24.e1–24.e20.
43. Poort LJ, Van Neck JW, Van der Wal KG. Sensory testing of inferior alveolar nerve injuries: a review of methods used in prospective studies. J Oral Maxillofac Surg. 2009;67(2):292–300.
44. Zuniga JR, Essick GK. A contemporary approach to the clinical evaluation of trigeminal nerve injuries. Oral Maxillofac Surg Clin North Am. 1992;4:353.
45. Cox B, Zuniga JR, Panchal N, Cheng J, Chhabra A. Magnetic resonance neurography in the management of peripheral trigeminal neuropathy: experience in a tertiary care centre. Eur Radiol. 2016;26(10):3392–400.
46. Dworkin RH, O'connor AB, Backonja M, et al. Pharmacologic management of neuropathic pain: evidence-based recommendations. Pain. 2007;132(3):237–51.
47. Dworkin RH, O'connor AB, Audette J, et al. Recommendations for the pharmacological management of neuropathic pain: an overview and literature update. Mayo Clin Proc. 2010;85(3 Suppl):S3–14.
48. Crider AB, Glaros AG. A meta-analysis of EMG biofeedback treatment of temporomandibular disorders. J Orofac Pain. 1999;13:29–37.
49. Phillips C, Essick G, Preisser JS, Turvey TA, Tucker M, Lin D. Sensory retraining after orthognathic surgery: effect on patients' perception of altered sensation. J Oral Maxillofac Surg. 2007;65(6):1162–73.
50. Kapur BM, Lala PK, Shaw JLV. Pharmacogenetics of chronic pain management. Clin Biochem. 2014;47:1169–87.
51. World Health Organization. http://www.who.int/cancer/palliative/painladder/en/. Accessed 05 Jan 2016.
52. Wiffen PJ, Derry S, Moore RA, Aldington D, Cole P, Rice A, Luna MD, Hamumen K, Haanpaa M, Kabo EA. Antiepilepsy drugs for neuropathic pain and fibromyalgia-an overview of Cochrane reviews. Cochrane Database Syst Rev. 2013;(11):CD010567.
53. Noble M, Treadwell JR, Tregear SJ, Coates VH, Wiffen PJ, Akafomo C, Schoelles KM. Long-term opioid management for chronic non-cancer pain. Cochrane Database Syst Rev. 2010;(1):CD006605
54. Gudin J. Assessment of extended-release opioid analgesics for the treatment of chronic pain. J Pain Palliat Care Pharmacother. 2013;27(1):49–61.
55. Chou R, Turner J, Devine E, Hansen R, Sullivan S, Blazina I, Dana T, Bougatsos C, Deyo R. The effectiveness and risks of long-term opioid therapy for chronic pain: a systematic review for a national institutes of health pathways to prevention workshop. Ann Intern Med. 2015;162:276–86.
56. Sehgal N, Colson J, Smith H. Chronic pain treatment with opioid analgesics: benefit versus harms of long-term therapy. Expert Rev Neurother. 2013;13:1201.
57. Vowles K, McEntee M, Julnes P, Frohe T, Ney J, Van der Goes D. Rates of opioid misuse, abuse, and addiction in chronic pain: a systematic review and data synthesis. Pain. 2015;156:569–76.
58. Bouloux GF. Use of opioids in long-term management of temporomandibular joint dysfunction. J Oral Maxillofac Surg. 2011;69:1885–91.

59. Nuckols T, Anderson L, Popescu I, Diamant A, Doyle B, Di Capua P, Chou R. Opioid prescribing: a systematic review and critical appraisal of guidelines for chronic pain. Ann Intern Med. 2014;160:38–47.
60. Deer T, Gunn J. Blood testing in chronic pain management. Pain Physician. 2015;18: E157–61.
61. Centers for disease control. http://www.cdc.gov/drugoverdose/data/overdose. Accessed 05 Jan 2016.
62. Ekholm O, Kurita G, Højsted J, Juel K, Sjøgren P. Chronic pain, opioid prescriptions, and mortality in Denmark: a population-based cohort study. Pain. 2014;155:2486.
63. Giummarra M, Gibson S, Allen A, Pichler A, Arnold C. Polypharmacy and chronic pain: harm exposure is not all about the opioids. Pain Med. 2015;16:472–9.
64. Provenzano D, Viscusi E. Rethinking the role of opioids in the outpatient management of chronic nonmalignant pain. Curr Med Res Opin. 2014;30:2051–62.
65. Hegmann K, Weiss M, Bowden K, Branco F, DuBrueler K, Els C, Mandel S, McKinney D, Miguel R, Mueller K, Nadig R, Schaffer M, Studt L, Talmage J, Travis R, Winters T, Thiese M, Harris J. ACOEM Practice Guidelines: Opioids for treatment of acute, subacute, chronic, and postoperative pain. J Occup Environ Med. 2014;56:e143–59.

Massive Hemorrhage

8

Eric J. Granquist and Peter D. Quinn

8.1 Introduction

Reconstruction of the temporomandibular joint (TMJ) requires careful preoperative planning, reasonable patient expectations, proper intraoperative technique, regimented postoperative physical therapy, close follow-up, and adequate pain management. The goals of TMJ reconstruction should include improved joint function and mastication, pain reduction, decreased morbidity, early rehabilitation, longevity of reconstruction, and cost consideration. Despite the best preoperative planning, intraoperative and postoperative complications will occur, and the temporomandibular joint surgeon should be well versed in the management and prevention of both common and catastrophic complications. The complication of massive hemorrhage is typically encountered intraoperatively but has been reported to occur up to 6 weeks postoperatively [1]. Along with several medium- and small-caliber arteries in close proximity to the temporomandibular joint, the parapharyngeal space and adjacent airway render even moderate swelling, a potential airway embarrassment. Therefore relatively easily managed complications such as an expanding hematoma may progress and compromise the airway or further complicate any potential re-intubation. Fortunately, the complication of massive hemorrhage is relatively

E.J. Granquist, DMD, MD (✉)
Director, Center for Temporomandibular Joint Disease, Oral and Maxillofacial Surgery and Pharmacology, University of Pennsylvania School of Dental Medicine,
Philadelphia, PA, USA
e-mail: eric.granquist@uphs.upenn.edu

P.D. Quinn, DMD, MD
Oral and Maxillofacial Surgery, University of Pennsylvania School of Dental Medicine,
Philadelphia, PA, USA

Vice Dean for Professional Services, University of Pennsylvania School of Medicine,
Philadelphia, PA, USA
e-mail: peter.quinn@uphs.upenn.edu

G.F. Bouloux (ed.), *Complications of Temporomandibular Joint Surgery*,
DOI 10.1007/978-3-319-51241-9_8

uncommon. Unfortunately, there is limited evidence-based literature to guide the prevention and management of massive hemorrhage. An understanding of the relevant anatomy, preoperative surgical planning, preventative surgical maneuvers, and techniques to control massive hemorrhage in the TMJ patient is paramount.

8.2 Anatomy

The head and neck, and temporomandibular joint in particular, have a rich vascular supply. This joint and its associated musculature are primarily supplied through branches of the external carotid artery. Collateral blood supply is also present due to the close proximity of contralateral vessels and communication between the external carotid artery and the intracranial internal carotid artery. Many nearby and overlying vessels may be encountered during a procedure involving the TMJ including the facial artery, temporal artery, temporal vein, facial vein, retromandibular vein, and external jugular vein (Fig. 8.1). These vessels are small caliber and generally easily accessed when injured. Inadvertent hemorrhage can be managed with minimal to moderate blood loss. The internal maxillary artery remains a potentially more concerning issue as access can be difficult through traditional approaches to the TMJ potentially resulting in massive hemorrhage.

The internal maxillary artery (IMAX) is classically divided into three portions. The branches of the first portion include deep auricular, anterior tympanic, middle meningeal, accessory meningeal, and inferior alveolar arteries. The second portion consists of the masseteric, pterygoid, deep temporalis, and buccal arteries, while the third portion enters the pterygopalatine fossa and includes the sphenopalatine, descending palatine, infraorbital, anterior superior alveolar, middle superior alveolar, posterior superior alveolar, artery of the pterygoid canal, and the pharyngeal arteries. It is the first portion of the internal maxillary artery that is at most risk for being injured and causing massive hemorrhage during a temporomandibular joint

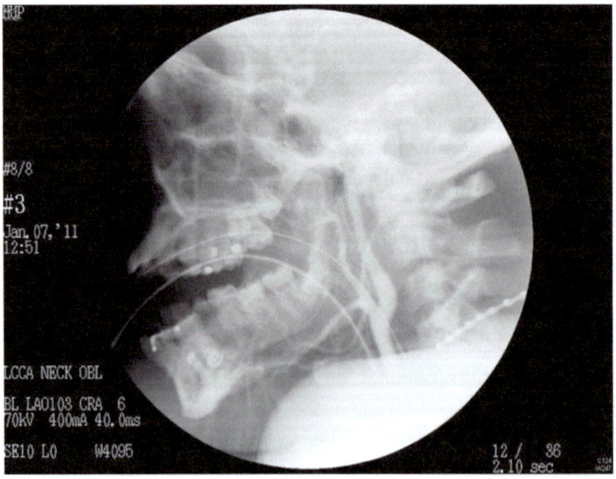

Fig. 8.1 Angiogram of the internal and external carotid arteries. This imaging was performed, and hemorrhage from the lingual artery was identified and the artery subsequently embolized. Note the fractured mandible

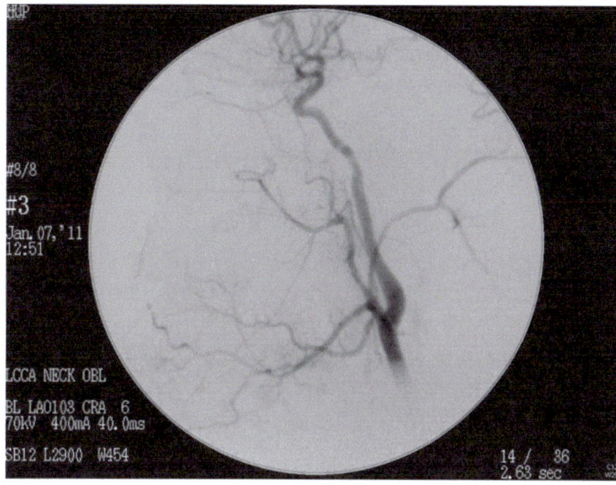

Fig. 8.2 Angiogram of the internal and external carotid arteries

procedure. The maxillary artery travels horizontally and medial to the neck of the mandible, with an intervening fat pad between the artery and the periosteum. Orbay, in a cadaveric study, found the mean distance between the artery and the medial border of the mandible in the subcondylar region to be 6.8 mm with a range of 4.06–8.47 mm [2]. The same authors found that the distance between the internal maxillary artery and the mandible ranges between 4.97 and 5.95 mm at the most inferior portion of the sigmoid notch, while others have reported a median distance of 2.94 mm [3]. The maxillary artery then courses anterior and medial, typically traveling superficial to the lateral pterygoid muscle, but this course is variable and it may run deep to the muscle as it continues toward the pterygopalatine fossa (Fig. 8.2).

The middle meningeal artery has also been reported to be a cause of massive hemorrhage from temporomandibular joint procedures [4]. The mean distance of the middle meningeal artery from the zygomatic arch was found to be 31 mm in a cadaveric study with a range of 21–44 mm [5]. In the same study, the artery was noted to be 2.4 mm anterior to the middle of the glenoid fossa with a range of −2–8 mm. Injury to this artery can be particularly catastrophic, as retraction of the vessel can result in a subdural hematoma [5]. In addition, the medial location of this vessel renders clamping or cautery difficult. As such, great care should be taken to avoid violation of the medial capsule during TMJ surgery.

The pterygoid venous plexus is a network of valveless veins located between the medial aspect of the temporal muscle and the lateral aspect of the pterygoid muscles. This plexus of veins communicates with the cavernous sinus superiorly and the retromandibular and facial vein inferiorly. The pterygoid venous plexus is situated within a fat pad [6]. Though uncommon, the operating surgeon may encounter this venous plexus in cases where the condyle has been displaced anteriorly or anteromedially such as in trauma or persistent dislocation. When bleeding is encountered in this region, it may at times become substantial. Isolation and ligation of individual vessels is very difficult, and controlling this venous bleed often requires packing and local measures in order to obtain hemostasis.

8.3 Preoperative Evaluation

Though rarely the etiology of difficult to control bleeding, patients undergoing surgery with the potential for massive hemorrhage should have a complete evaluation for congenital or acquired coagulopathies [1]. This includes review of the patients' family history for bleeding disorders, a focused review of systems discussing bleeding or easy bruising, experiences with past surgeries, and coagulation labs including a complete blood count, platelet function, prothrombin time (PT/INR), and partial thrombin time (PTT). The use of oral anticoagulation medications should be sought including aspirin, warfarin, adenosine diphosphate receptor inhibitors (clopidogrel, prasugrel, ticagrelor, ticlopidine), as well as directly acting anticoagulants (dabigatran, rivaroxaban, apixaban, and edoxaban). Additional laboratory tests to quantitate the effect of the direct factor Xa inhibitors are available but are not routinely used. Any alterations in laboratory values, review of systems, family history, or bleeding difficulties with prior surgeries should prompt consideration for a hematology consultation. Patients with a known bleeding disorder warrant close communication and planning with the patient's hematologist.

In cases of ankylosis or previous surgeries where altered anatomy may be encountered, a CT angiogram (CTA) should be considered (Fig. 8.3a, b). This allows for the evaluation and visualization of vessels that may be encountered intraoperatively, where known anatomic landmarks may not be useful to the operating surgeon. Scarring or immobility of the mandible, secondary to ankylosis or multiple procedures, may limit access to deeper structures. As such, vessels, which are at increased risk of injury and may be difficult to access and ligate, can be identified. In cases where there is intimate involvement of the vasculature and mandible, selective embolization may be considered preoperatively [7]. The utilization and benefit of CTA in the preoperative evaluation of patients with ankylosis of the TMJ has been previously reported [8]. In this study Susarla presented five subjects who underwent CTA prior to resection. In three of the five cases, evidence of intimate association between the ankylotic mass and the vasculature was found, necessitating selective embolization. The authors reported a significant reduction in blood loss during surgery when embolization was performed compared to surgical procedures performed without embolization. No complications from the embolization procedure were reported. At our institution, selective preoperative embolization typically occurs the day prior to the procedure with 24 h of intensive care unit (ICU) observation and hourly neurologic examination. Surgery has been performed up to 3 days

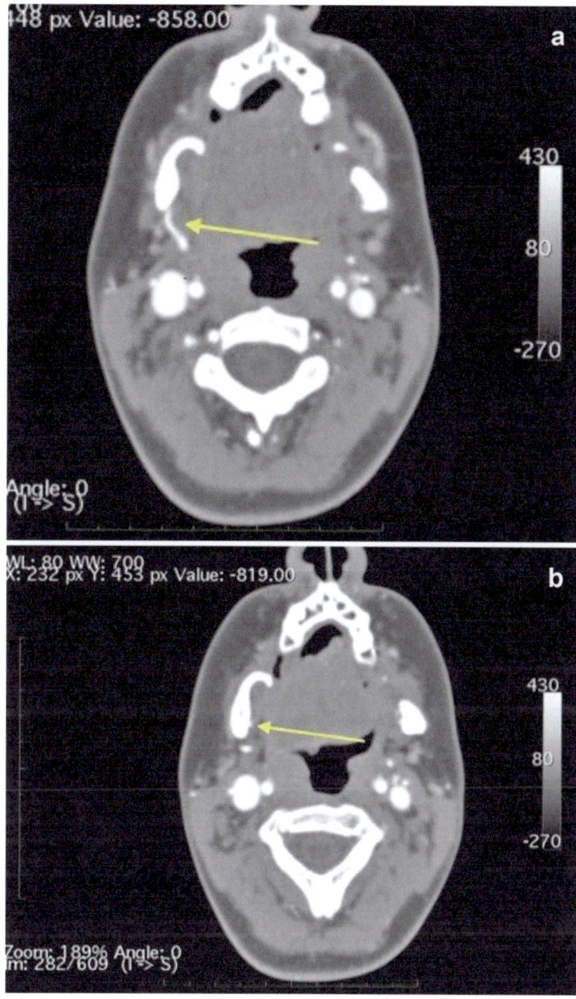

Fig. 8.3 (**a**, **b**) CT angiogram of the mandible with axial views. *Yellow arrow* identifies the internal maxillary artery in the retromandibular fossa (**a**) and as the artery courses medially along the inner aspect of the mandible (**b**)

post-embolization. A number of agents can be used to embolize the vessel including gelatin sponge, glue, or small metal coils [7, 9]. Selective embolization is not without complication and may include skin necrosis, migration of the coils or embolic agents, blindness, and neurologic deficits [7]. It is also worth noting that CTA and embolization have large associated contrast dye loads, which may result in acute kidney injury. These risks, along with the risks of intraoperative hemorrhage, should be discussed with the patient before proceeding with this preoperative intervention (Figs. 8.4 and 8.5).

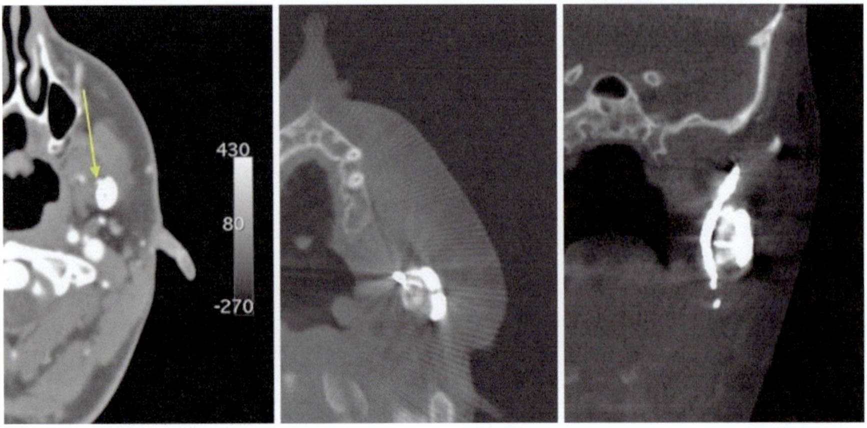

Fig. 8.4 CT angiogram of the mandible with axial views (*left*), with *yellow arrow* identifying the internal maxillary artery. Postoperative images of the same patient (*middle* and *right*) demonstrating selective embolization prior to total joint reconstruction. Note the close proximity of the prosthesis, osteotomies, and artery in this patient

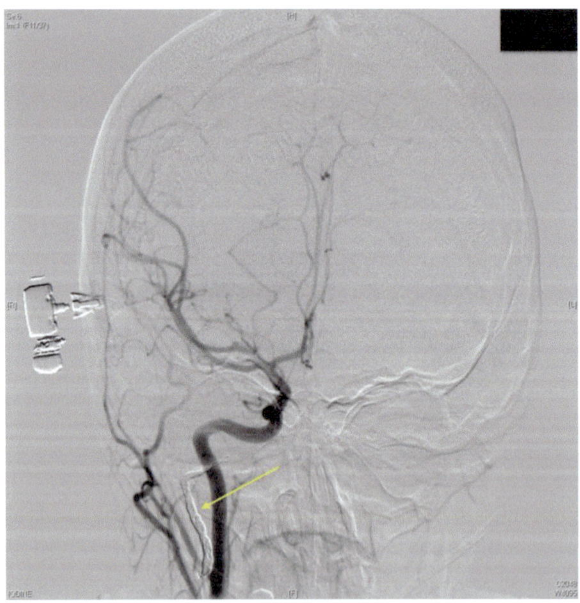

Fig. 8.5 Angiogram of the right head and neck arteries. The *yellow arrow* identifies the embolized right internal maxillary artery

The potential for intraoperative bleeding should also alert the surgeon and anesthesiologist to the potential need for blood transfusion. A type and screen is strongly encouraged prior to the procedure to avoid any delay should a transfusion become necessary.

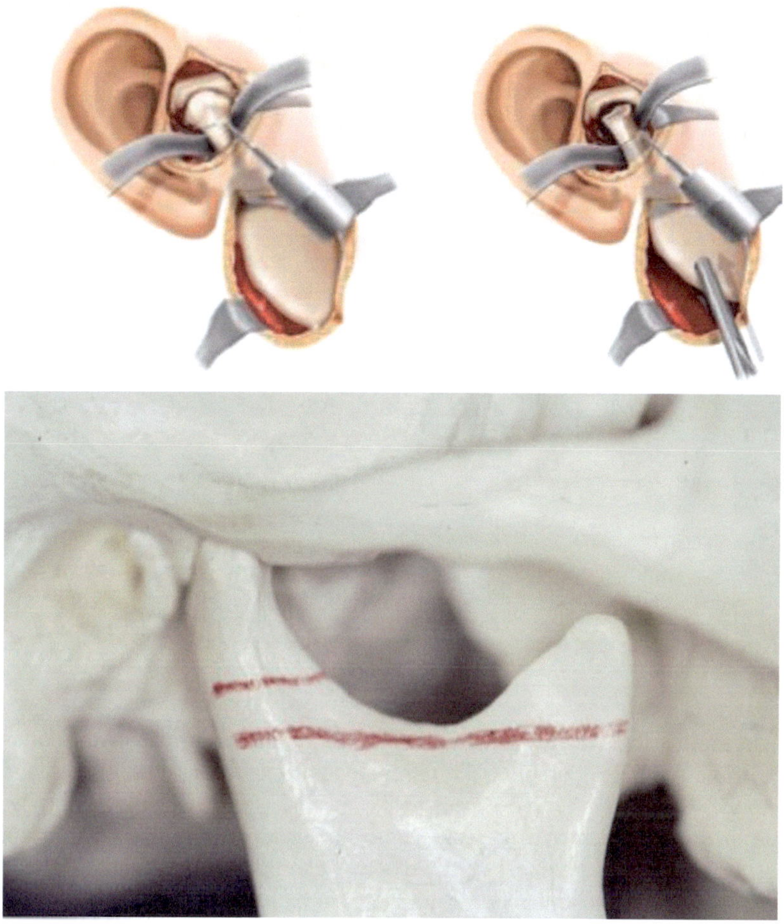

Fig. 8.6 *Upper left* and *right diagram* depicting the two-step condylectomy. Note on the upper left, a bone holding forceps is used to access the mandible through the neck incision and superiorly reposition the bone. *Bottom image* shows the initial osteotomy for the condylectomy (*upper red line*) and the final osteotomy (*lower red line*)

8.4 Surgical Techniques to Avoid Vessel Injury

Condylectomy of the TMJ provides the greatest opportunity to encounter excessive hemorrhage as the internal maxillary runs nearest the mandible along the condyle and sigmoid notch and often parallels the planned osteotomy. As such, great care should be taken when performing osteotomies along the neck of the condyle or near the sigmoid notch. One technique developed to minimize injury while performing the

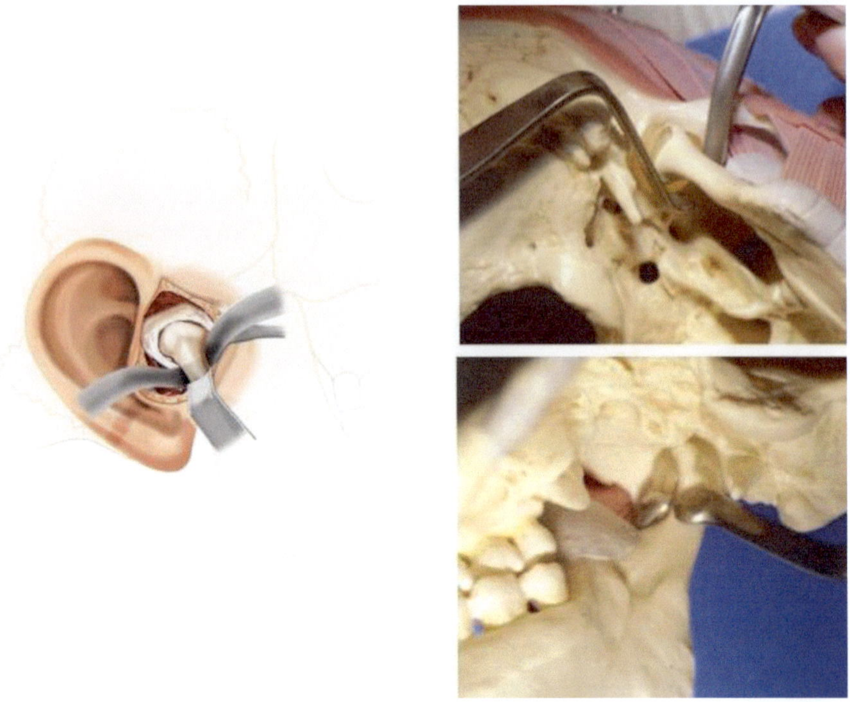

Fig. 8.7 Diagram and image showing the positioning of the Dunn-Dautrey condylar neck retractors. Note on the lower right image the medial position of the retractors

condylectomy is the two-step osteotomy (Fig. 8.6). Prior to performing the condylectomy, it is essential to complete the retromandibular incision prior to the condylar osteotomy. This ensures rapid access to the medial aspect of the mandible with a simple finger dissection and pressure with immediate hemostasis. It also provides access to the terminal branches of the external carotid, in cases where difficult-to-control bleeding is encountered. Furthermore, in patients with ankylosis where the risk of hemorrhage is high, consideration may be given for identification and isolation of the external carotid artery prior to the osteotomy although ligation of this vessel and its branches may not arrest bleeding due to a significant collateral blood supply [10].

Once the retromandibular incision and access to the ramus of the mandible are completed, the endaural (or preauricular) access to the lateral portion of neck of the condyle is initiated. A No. 15 blade is then used to place a vertical incision through the periosteum of the neck of the condyle. A freer can then be used to carefully develop a subperiosteal pocket around the condylar neck. Two Dunn-Dautrey retractors are carefully placed in this subperiosteal pocket, allowing the contents medial to the mandible to be well protected (Fig. 8.7). Once the neck of the condyle is fully exposed, a one-millimeter fissure bur is used to perform the condylectomy. The use of a piezoelectric saw has also been described to minimize soft tissue injury, but with well-placed retractors within the surgical field, the use of this device may be unnecessary [11]. If adequate protection of the soft tissue medial to the ankylotic mass is not possible, the use of the piezoelectric saw may be a reasonable measure. The osteotomy with a 1 mm side cutting fissure bur is performed by first starting at the midpoint of the condylar neck, sparing the medial cortex. The cut is then extended both anteriorly and posteriorly toward the Dunn-Dautrey retractors. A T-bar osteotome is then used to complete the final 5–10% of the osteotomy. The condyle is then grasped with a bone holding forceps, and the lateral pterygoid is then carefully dissected free. At this point, significant bleeding may occur, and the surgeon should be ready to control any hemorrhage with the aid of hemostatic agents. With the condyle removed, the mandible is superiorly repositioned by grasping the inferior border through the retromandibular incision with a bone holding forceps. This allows for the second osteotomy, at the level of the inferior portion of the sigmoid notch, to occur at a safer distance from the internal maxillary artery. This "second cut" is necessary to allow for adequate room for the placement of an alloplastic fossa implant and/or to create a "critical size defect" to minimize re-ankylosis.

8.5 Intraoperative Management of Massive Hemorrhage

When the surgeon encounters massive hemorrhage, ideally proximal and distal control is established with ligation of the injured vessel. Unfortunately, secondary to vessel contraction or access, this is not always possible. The first priority should be to slow or stop the blood loss in order to allow for visualization and assessment of the hemorrhage. This can be accomplished through direct pressure with packing of the wound. Alternatively placing a digit through the neck incision, along the posterior aspect of the mandible, and concurrently a second digit directly through the preauricular incision can place bimanual digital pressure on the internal maxillary artery. This may slow the bleeding and allow the nursing staff to obtain additional hemostatic agents, inform anesthesia of the hemorrhage and possible need for blood transfusion, as well as give the surgeon additional time to evaluate the situation. Once the hemorrhage has diminished either through packing or direct pressure, identification of the injured vessel and ligation and/or cautery should be attempted. If this fails, utilization of thrombin-saturated packing or a collagen-based hemostatic agent packed in the wound should be attempted. Cillo et al. described a case of successfully managing a middle meningeal and superficial temporal artery hemorrhage with the use of FloSeal™[1], a gelatin-based network with collagen and topical thrombin [4]. The use of electrocautery or vasoconstrictors such as epinephrine may be considered but is less successful in massive hemorrhage. If all local measures have been exhausted, the surgeon has several options: the wound can be packed and the procedure aborted, the external carotid artery can be ligated, or the patient can be taken to interventional radiology for angiography and embolization. If packing of the wound is chosen, a minimum of 3 days is generally recommended while in the ICU with subsequent

[1] ™Baxter, Fremont, CA, USA

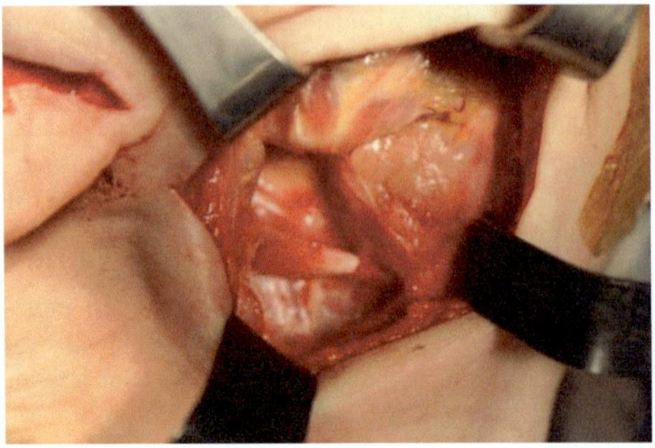

Fig. 8.8 Modified retromandibular approach to the mandible. The dissection to the level of the posterior digastric (shown) should occur prior to the condylectomy. This ensures rapid access to the vasculature should a difficult-to-control hemorrhage occur

packing removal in the OR, either with or without ligation of the external carotid artery or embolization. Rosenberg et al. evaluated the effects of ligation of the external carotid artery and blood flow in baboons, given their close anatomic vascular similarity [12]. They found a 40% decrease in blood flow with ligation above the origin of the lingual artery, a 73% reduction with ligation above the facial artery, and a 99% reduction with ligation above the posterior auricular artery, although the more distal the ligation, the more technically difficult it is to perform. It is important to note that 24% of the mean flow occurred from the distal segment from collateral blood flow. Due to collateral flow, their recommendations for control of hemorrhage from the internal maxillary artery included ligation of the external carotid in the retromandibular fossa along with ligation of the superficial temporal artery. Yen investigated the flow in the maxillary artery after ligation of the external carotid artery in dogs, with similar results [13]. Blood flow from the IMAX was reduced by 61% with ligation of the external carotid above the lingual artery and 71% with ligation above the facial artery. Of note, there was an 81% reduction of blood flow with multiple ligations of the external carotid along with the lingual, facial, and occipital arteries, reducing retrograde blood flow. It was felt that blood flow could have been further reduced had the superficial temporal artery been ligated as well. The same authors reported on four cases of hemorrhage from the internal maxillary artery treated with multiple points of ligation along the external carotid artery [14]. Although ligation of the external carotid artery when performed near the site of hemorrhage is often successful, subsequent selective embolization becomes impossible if the ligation fails to control bleeding [10] (Figs. 8.8 and 8.9).

In summary, avoidance of massive hemorrhage requires careful preoperative planning. Considerations should be given for preoperative CTA in patients with massive ankylosis, severely altered anatomy, or a history of multiple operations and subsequent trismus. If intimate involvement of the bone and vasculature is found, the surgeon should decide whether selective immobilization or isolation of the

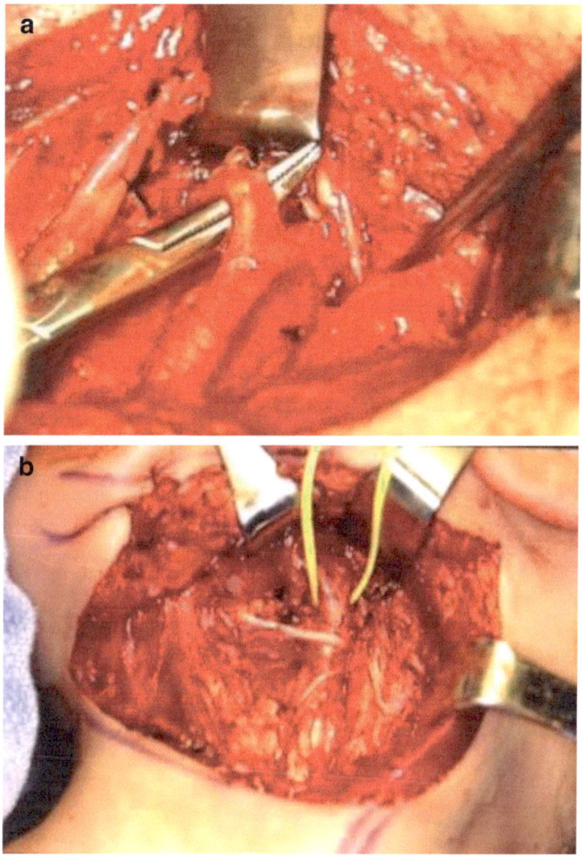

Fig. 8.9 (**a, b**) Isolation of the external carotid artery (**a, b**). On the right, note the hypoglossal nerve (**b**)

external carotid artery is indicated. Intraoperatively, every effort should be made to avoid violating the periosteum of the medial aspect of the condylar neck or medial capsule of the temporomandibular joint. This can be accomplished with well-placed retractors or the use of a piezoelectric saw. Despite the best planning efforts, avoidance of inadvertent vessel injury is not always possible, and all members of the operating room team should be prepared to manage significant hemorrhage.

References

1. Lanigan DT, Hey J, West RA. Hemorrhage following mandibular osteotomies: a report of 21 cases. J Oral Maxillofac Surg. 1991;49:713.
2. Orbay H, et al. Maxillary artery: anatomical landmarks and relationship with the mandibular subcondyle. Plast Reconstr Surg. 2007;120:1865.
3. Balcioglu HA, et al. A Morphometric study of the Maxillary Artery and Lingula in Relation to Mandibular Ramus Osteotomies and TMJ Surgery. Eur J Dent. 2010;4:167.

4. Cillo JE, Sinn D, Truelson JM. Management of middle meningeal and superficial temporal artery hemorrhage from total temporomandibular replacement surgery with a gelatin-based hemostatic agent. J Craniofac Surg. 2005;16:309.
5. Talebzadeh N, Rosenstein TP, Pogrel MA. Anatomy of the structures medial to the temporomandibular joint. Oral Surg Oral Med Oral Pathol Oral Radiol Endod. 1999;88:674.
6. Isolan GR, Rowe R, Al-Mefty O. Microanatomy and surgical approaches to the infratemporal fossa: an anaglyphic three-dimensional stereoscopic printing study. Skull Base. 2007;17:285.
7. Peoples JR, Herbosa EG, Dion J. Management of internal maxillary artery hemorrhage from temporomandibular joint surgery via selective embolization. J Oral Maxillofac Surg. 1988;46:1005.
8. Susarla SM, et al. Role of computed tomographic angiography in treatment of patients with temporomandibular joint ankylosis. J Oral Maxillofac Surg. 2014;72:267.
9. Elahi MM, et al. Therapeutic embolization in the treatment of intractable epistaxis. Arch Otolaryngol Head Neck Surg. 1995;121:65.
10. Bouloux GF, Perciaccante VJ. Massive hemorrhage during oral and maxillofacial surgery: ligation of the external carotid artery or embolization? J Oral Maxillofac Surg. 2009;67:1547.
11. Jose A, et al. Piezoelectric osteoarthrectomy for management of ankylosis of the temporomandibular joint. Br J Oral Maxillofac Surg. 2014;52:624.
12. Rosenberg I, Austin C, Wright PG, King RE. The effect of experimental ligation of the external carotid artery and its major branches on hemorrhage from the maxillary artery. Int J Oral Surg. 1982;11:251.
13. Yen NT. Effect of multiple ligations of the external carotid artery and its branches on blood flow in the internal maxillary artery in dogs. J Oral Maxillofac Surg. 1994;52:849.
14. Yen NT. Hemorrhage of the initial part of the internal maxillary artery treated by multiple ligations: report of four cases. Oral Maxillofac Surg. 1994;52:1066.

Diagnosis and Management of TMJ Heterotopic Bone and Ankylosis

9

Larry M. Wolford

9.1 Introduction

Temporomandibular joint (TMJ) heterotopic bone refers to calcifications that develop in and around areas of the joint that are normally void of the bone. The development of heterotopic bone within the confines of a joint or in the surrounding area can cause joint dysfunction, pain, as well as progression to ankylosis. Temporomandibular joint ankylosis is a condition where the condyle is fused to the fossa by bony or fibrotic tissues creating a debilitating condition that can interfere with jaw function, mastication, speech, oral hygiene, growth and development, breathing, and normal life activities and cause pain. There are numerous surgical techniques that have been proposed to manage heterotopic bone and TMJ ankylosis with varying outcomes reported. The most common complications following the treatment of ankylosis are limited jaw function, pain, and re-ankylosis.

9.2 Etiology

The formation of TMJ heterotopic bone and ankylosis is most commonly caused from trauma but can also be related to inflammation or bone growth stimulation related to various TMJ pathologies such as infection, reactive arthritis, osteoarthritis, inflammatory conditions, connective tissue/autoimmune diseases (e.g., juvenile idiopathic arthritis, rheumatoid arthritis, psoriatic arthritis, ankylosing spondylitis, scleroderma, etc.), endocrine and metabolic disorders, multiply operated joints,

L.M. Wolford, DMD
Department of Oral and Maxillofacial Surgery, Texas A&M University College of Dentistry, Dallas, TX, USA

Department of Orthodontics, Texas A&M University College of Dentistry, Dallas, TX, USA
e-mail: lwolford@swbell.net

G.F. Bouloux (ed.), *Complications of Temporomandibular Joint Surgery*,
DOI 10.1007/978-3-319-51241-9_9

foreign-body giant-cell reaction, repeated injections of medications into the TMJ (i.e., steroids), as well as unsuccessful previous TMJ surgeries including failed TMJ autogenous grafts and alloplastic implants. Heterotopic bone in the initial phase may be asymptomatic, but with further development can create pain, decrease range of motion, and may lead to ankylosis. A variable amount of fibrosis and reactive tissue are normally associated with heterotopic bone, thereby worsening the adverse effects.

Bleeding into a joint by trauma or a surgical procedure as well as the presence of dead space following extensive TMJ debridement or reconstruction with autogenous bone or total joint prosthesis can lead to blood clot formation in the joint area, with subsequent organization. Pluripotential cells can then migrate into the area and differentiate into fibroblasts and osteoblasts, with deposition of collagen and then bone, respectively. This results in the potential for developing heterotopic bone and ankylosis. In excessively fibrotic joints, there is also a decrease in tissue vascularity with a resultant decrease in oxygen tension in the surrounding tissue. This can lead to the transformation of fibrous tissue into cartilage and bone with potential for ankylosis [1]. Temporomandibular joint ankylosis can be even more devastating in growing patients resulting in a profound dentofacial deformity in addition to jaw dysfunction and malocclusion.

9.3 Diagnosis

The diagnosis of TMJ heterotopic bone and ankylosis is usually determined by clinical examination and imaging studies such as CT scans, cone beam CT (CBCT), magnetic resonance imaging (MRI), and the three-dimensional reconstruction of images or stereolithic models. It is important to know the patient's TMJ history relative to age of onset, etiology, previous TMJ treatment, present age, current and past symptoms, medical history and conditions, other joint involvement, allergies, and history of hypersensitivity to metals particularly those used in TMJ total joint prostheses. Guidelines on patient evaluation and treatment for combined TMJ and orthognathic surgery have been previously published [2–8]. Patients with TMJ pathology resulting in heterotopic bone or ankylosis may present with facial symmetry and balance, or they can present with a retruded mandible with the potential for maxillary involvement and facial asymmetry. Patients may have a profound limited opening if the ankylosing bone is predominately cortical in nature or can have moderate opening if the bone is softer with a more cancellous bone composition. In unilateral cases, there may be deviation toward the ipsilateral side with jaw opening as the contralateral side may maintain translation. Patients may have a coexisting dentofacial deformity that was preexisting or developed as a result of the original TMJ injury and pathology or from the ankylosis.

Radiographic imaging may show heterotopic bone in and around the joint area and is best seen on CBCT imaging (Fig. 9.1a, b). The ability of CBCT scans to identify newly developing heterotopic bone may be difficult with the presence of total joint prostheses due to scatter. A medical-grade CT scan is better than CBCT for identifying heterotopic bone around a TJP because of the higher resolution and

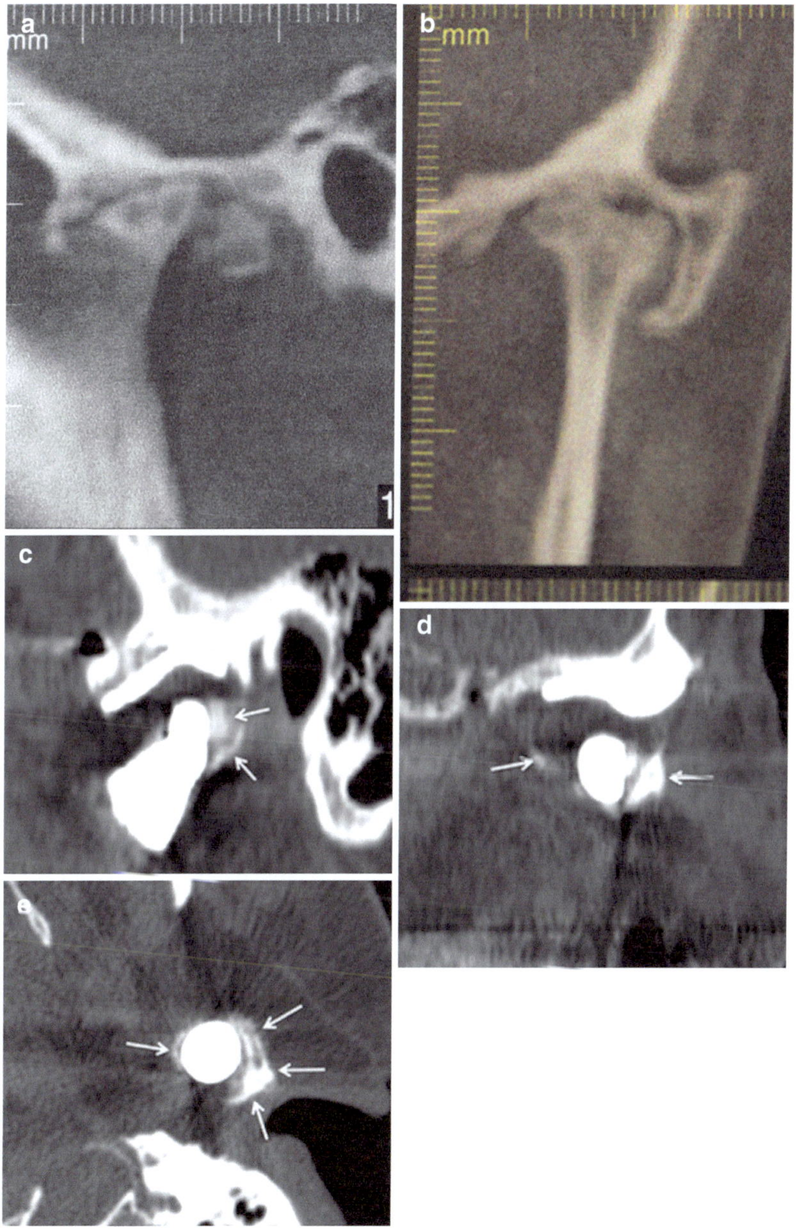

Fig. 9.1 (**a, b**) 22-year-old female with history of adolescent internal condylar resorption (AICR). She had multiple steroid injections into the TMJ resulting in heterotopic bone formation. (**a**) CBCT left TMJ sagittal view and (**b**) coronal view. (**c–e**) 53-year-old female patient with multiple previous surgeries including failed Proplast-Teflon material. Patient was reconstructed with a custom total joint prostheses, but developed heterotopic bone around the prosthesis in reaction to the residual Proplast-Teflon materials, at 10 years postsurgery, creating severe pain and limited jaw function. (**c**) CT scan left sagittal view with *white arrows* pointing to the heterotopic bone, (**d**) coronal view, (**e**) axial view

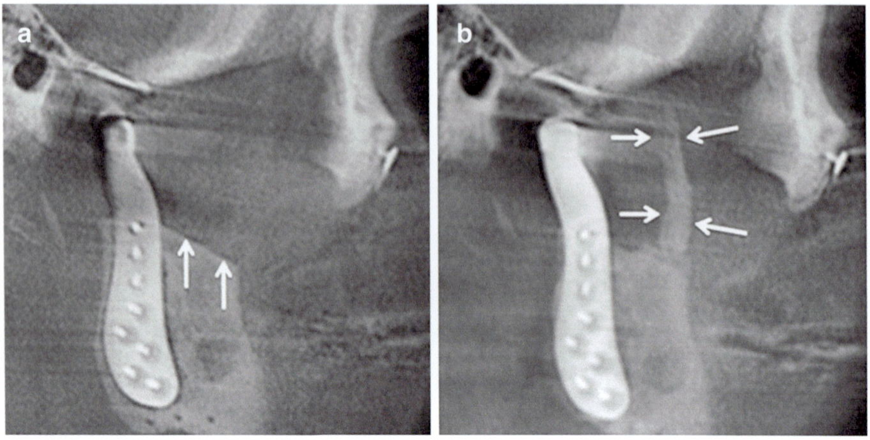

Fig. 9.2 (**a, b**) Coronoid area heterotopic bone formation; 15-year-old female with history of juvenile idiopathic arthritis treated in a single surgery with bilateral TMJ Concepts prostheses, maxillary osteotomies, TMJ fat grafts, and coronoidectomies. (**a**) Right TMJ immediate postsurgery showing level of coronoidectomy (*white arrows*). (**b**) 4 months postsurgery; patient developed heterotopic bone in the original coronoid process area (*white arrows*)

quality (Fig. 9.1c–e). However, when the previous TMJ reconstruction is autogenous, either imaging technique will usually be diagnostic. Heterotopic bone most commonly develops around the TMJ on the medial side, followed by posterior, anterior, and lateral aspects. Heterotopic bone and ankylosis can also develop in the coronoid area (Fig. 9.2a, b). This may require a different approach for management as compared with heterotopic bone associated directly with the TMJ.

When TMJ bony ankylosis occurs during the growing years, it can adversely affect jaw growth and development. The common clinical and radiographic characteristics of TMJ ankylosis include decreased jaw mobility and function, decreased growth on the involved side(s), facial asymmetry if unilateral involvement with the mandible shifted toward the ipsilateral side, retruded mandible, a Class II occlusion, high occlusal plane angle facial morphology, and imaging evidence of bony ankylosis at the condyle/fossa area.

9.4 Treatment Options

The ultimate goal in treatment of TMJ heterotopic bone formation and ankylosis is to return the patient to normal function with stable skeletal and occlusal results, correct associated facial and occlusal deformity, decrease pain, and prevent redevelopment of heterotopic bone and re-ankylosis.

Multiple surgical options have been proposed to treat TMJ ankylosis including gap arthroplasty, interpositional arthroplasty, and autogenous or alloplastic total joint reconstruction. Autogenous tissues that have been used after gap arthroplasty include ear cartilage, temporalis muscle flap, dermis, and fat. Some alloplastic materials such as Proplast Teflon®[1], Silastic®[2], and metal fossa liners have also been used, but with higher failure rates [9, 10].

Total joint reconstruction can be divided into autogenous tissue replacement such as costochondral (CCG) and sternoclavicular grafts (SCG) [11–14] or alloplastic total joint prosthesis (TJP) reconstruction. The CCG has had mixed results in TMJ reconstruction [15–18]. Costochondral grafts and SCG grafts used for ankylosis in adults or children have common postoperative complications including re-ankylosis (resorption, no growth, overgrowth) [19, 20], fracture, and pain. Sternoclavicular grafts have growth potential for younger patients similar to the mandibular condyle, and a section of the SCG articular disc can be harvested with the SCG providing the potential for better function, but re-ankylosis is still a significant risk [14].

Wolford and colleagues [21–33], Mercuri and colleagues [34–44], and others [45–47] have validated the successful use of TMJ Concepts™[3] patient-fitted TJP for TMJ reconstruction. The TMJ Concepts devices are computer-assisted-designed/computer-assisted-manufactured (CAD/CAM) devices, designed and manufactured to fit the specific anatomical, functional, and esthetic requirements of each specific patient. Temporomandibular joint TJP by themselves may not prevent heterotopic bone development and re-ankylosis, particularly in the presence of significant inflammatory disease and previous ankylosis [27, 48].

9.4.1 Nonsurgical Options

In the orthopedic experience, various pharmacologic agents, most notably indomethacin and etidronate, have been used with varying success in preventing heterotopic bone in hip and knee TJP reconstruction [49, 50]. Pharmacologic therapy has been suggested for use after TMJ TJP reconstruction, but no data exists regarding its effectiveness. Radiation treatment of the operated area within 4 days of prosthetic hip reconstruction is now a common practice and appears to offer an effective means of preventing heterotopic bone formation in orthopedics. However, local radiation of the TMJ raises concerns regarding potential adverse effects on adjacent vital structures. The use of postoperative radiation (10Gy) following CCG, gap arthroplasty, or debridement of heterotopic bone has been shown to still result in heterotopic bone in 33–50% of cases [51, 52].

9.4.2 Gap Arthroplasty and Grafts

Various techniques have been used to treat TMJ ankylosis including gap arthroplasty with or without tissue grafts and flaps. The long-term functional results after gap arthroplasty and interpositional grafting have been shown to be comparable to those obtained through use of other treatments [53]. However, the incidence of

[1] ®Vitek Inc., Houston, TX.

[2] ®Dow-Corning, Midland, MO.

[3] ™TMJ Concepts, Ventura, CA.

re-ankylosis with gap arthroplasty does appear to be higher than with CCG [54]. An additional problem with gap arthroplasty either with or without an interposing tissue is the vertical stability of the mandible and the occlusion.

Topazian compared gap arthroplasty with interpositional arthroplasty in TMJ ankylosis surgery and found interpositional arthroplasty to provide more favorable results [55]. The use of temporalis myofascial flaps and dermal grafts also appear to produce satisfactory results [56]. Similar results have been reported with the use of dermis-fat grafts [57–59]. The pedicled vascularized temporalis myofascial flap continues to be a relatively predictable and stable interpositional graft following gap arthroplasty. The ability of this flap to prevent heterotopic bone is less clear in part due to the lack of a critical-sized defect with this flap.

Concomitant use of CCG and the temporalis myofascial flap has also been reported to be successful in maintaining the occlusion with good functional outcomes and decreased pain [60–62]. The disadvantages of CCG are the poor quality of medullary and cortical bone, the possibility of resorption or infection, bone flexibility, elasticity that may cause the graft to be deformed, possible separation of the cartilage from the bone, and occasional fractures. Furthermore, the inherent growth potential of CCG can result in unpredictable growth.

9.4.3 Fat Grafts

The first reported use of autologous fat graft placement into the TMJ for the treatment of ankylosis is more than 100 years old [63, 64]. Wolford reported a technique of placing autogenous fat grafts around TJP to prevent postsurgical heterotopic bone and fibrosis development in 1992 [48]. The rationale for placing autologous fat grafts around the TMJ TJP was to obliterate the dead space surrounding the prosthesis, thus preventing the formation and subsequent organization of a blood clot. Creating this physical barrier, the fat grafts serve to reduce the differentiation of pluripotential cells and prevent the formation of extensive fibrosis and heterotopic calcification. Fat grafts have been shown to inhibit osteogenesis in other bone defects [65]. The fate of fat grafts has also been described with the graft going through a period of initial breakdown of fat cells, followed by revascularization, resulting in normal appearing fat, although a smaller volume than originally grafted [66]. The early and adequate revascularization of autogenous fat grafts for maintenance of graft volume and for the production of adipocyte-derived angiogenic peptides such as vascular endothelial growth factor (VEGF) and leptin which are important for graft survival and volume maintenance has been reported [67, 68]. However, following free fat grafting, the fat shows features of ischemia with adipocytes releasing lipid and dedifferentiating to pre-adipocytes. After revascularization, the pre-adipocytes begin to absorb lipid and develop into mature adipocytes with the fat grafts almost normal at 6 months [69].

The use of fat grafts around TMJ TJP has been shown to be superior to no fat grafting when evaluating both maximum incisal opening, the development of heterotopic bone, and re-ankylosis [31, 48, 70–72]. The importance of using fat grafts to prevent heterotopic bone may be even more important in those patients who have had Proplast-Teflon and Silastic implants given the increase inflammatory response

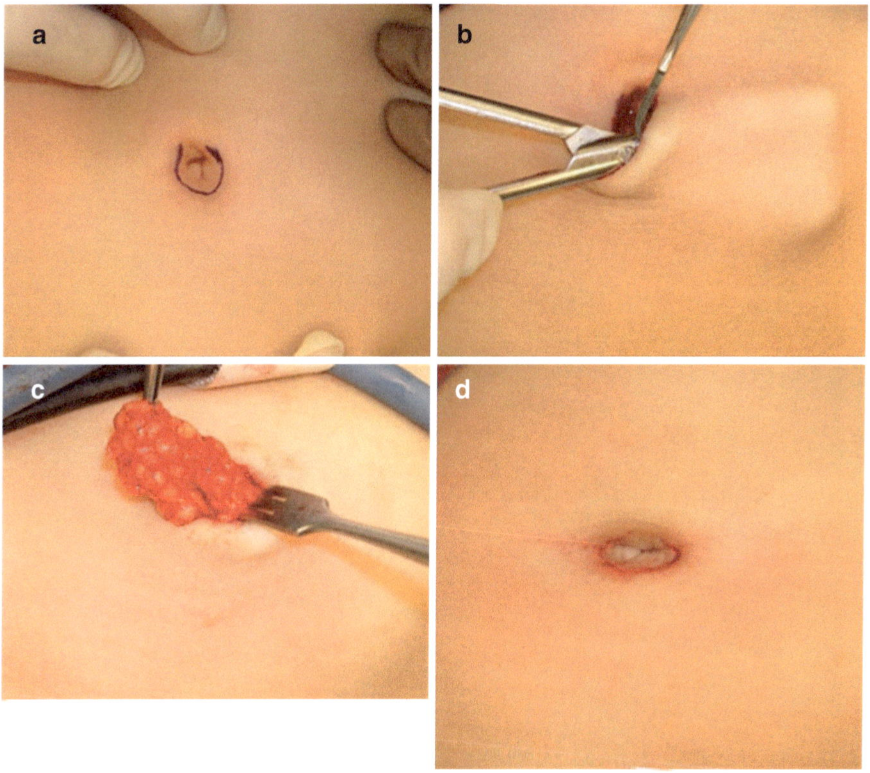

Fig. 9.3 (**a**) Umbilical incision outlined. (**b**) Following incision, a superficial and deeper dissection is completed. (**c**) Fat being delivered. (**d**) Incision closed

within the TMJ tissues and the likelihood of heterotopic bone formation [26, 27]. Despite the apparent benefit to the use of fat grafts in preventing heterotopic bone, complications at the donor site have been reported to occur in about 10% of patients with abdominal cysts and seroma formation the most common.

The ultimate fate of the transplanted fat around the TMJ is unknown. Studies of fat transplantation to other anatomic areas show a variable amount of resorption, with a decrease in volume ranging from 20 to 75% [73, 74]. As an adjunct to TMJ prosthetic joint reconstruction, the ultimate resorption of a portion of the graft may not be detrimental to the result. If the formation of the initial hematoma, fibrosis, and reactive tissue can be prevented by placement of the fat grafts, there may be reduced incidence of complications.

The most common donor site for fat harvesting is the abdomen, where there is usually abundant or at least adequate fat for most cases. The most common approaches the author uses include the supra-pubic incision, the umbilical or trans-naval incision (Fig. 9.3a–d), or approach through a preexisting scar (e.g., C-section, hysterectomy, appendectomy, abdominoplasty). However, the fat can be harvested from almost any fat source including the buttock, thigh, buccal fat pad, or breast. Following fat harvest, good hemostasis of the donor site is required and a pressure dressing applied

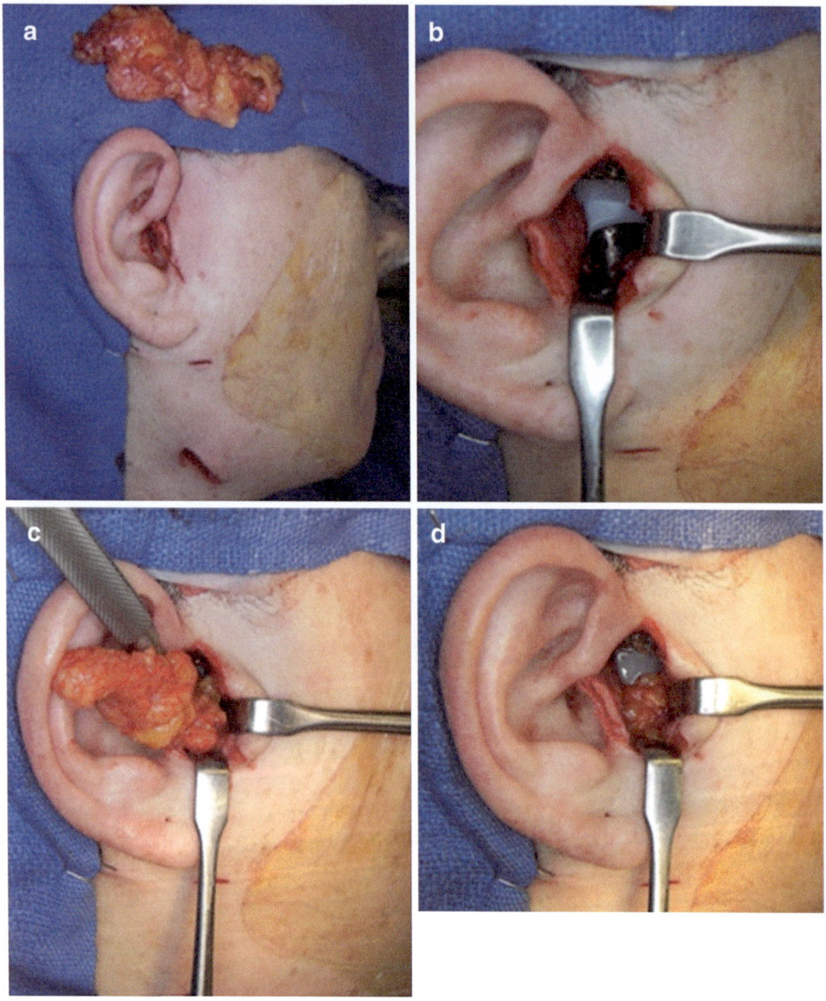

Fig. 9.4 (**a**) Harvested fat ready for implantation. (**b**) Total joint prosthesis visualized. (**c**) Fat packed around prosthesis medially, posterior, anterior, and lateral. (**d**) Fat packing completed

along with an abdominal binder (for abdominal donor site) for 3–4 days postsurgery to prevent hematoma or seroma formation. If adequate hemostasis cannot be achieved, then a drain with negative pressure may be indicated for a few days.

Fat grafts are harvested just prior to graft placement, requiring only about 20 min of additional surgical time. However, some surgeons may prefer to have two surgical teams working concurrently so the overall operation is not prolonged. It is not recommended to harvest the fat grafts prior to beginning the TMJ reconstruction as this would require the grafts to be "on the table" for an extended time period, likely to result in significant loss of graft viability. It will usually take a minimum of 4 h to prepare the TMJs and place the prostheses in bilateral cases, before the fat grafts can be placed (Fig. 9.4a–d). Therefore, procuring the fat graft just prior to placement will maximize graft viability, an important factor for graft survival. We recommend harvesting the fat graft in bulk and not procuring with liposuction as this can severely damage the fat cells providing poorer quality of results with greater fat resorption.

9.4.4 Ankylosis in Autogenous Reconstruction Versus Total Joint Prostheses (TJP)

The incidence of re-ankylosis following joint reconstruction with CCG or SCG when not using a fat graft has been reported to be 100 and 75%, respectively [75]. Furthermore, the CCG and SCG resulted in excessive growth or relapse, while SCG and TJP reconstruction with fat grafting resulted in stability and no re-ankylosis. Long-term surgical stability and improved subjective and objective outcomes have also been reported in patients undergoing maxillomandibular advancement with TJP when compared to CCG and SCG [76]. The incidence of complications requiring additional surgery has also been reported to be significantly higher in autogenous reconstruction compared to TJP [77].

9.5 Surgical Protocol for Managing Heterotopic Bone

A complication that may be encountered following TMJ reconstruction with autogenous tissues or alloplastic TJP involves heterotopic bone formation in and around the TMJ. This can result in pain and decreased function. When heterotopic bone develops around an autogenous TMJ graft and is symptomatic, the most predictable treatment protocol includes removal of the autogenous graft and heterotopic bone, reconstruction with a total joint prosthesis, and placing fat graft around the articulating area of the prosthesis. Heterotopic bone that forms around a TJP is best managed by debridement and removal of the heterotopic bone and placing a fat graft around the articulating area of the prosthesis. The debridement can usually be done without removal of the prosthesis although if needed the condyle component can be removed to improve access, re-sterilized, and secured back to the ramus with larger screws. The fossa component should not be removed as this would require a new fossa prosthesis as this component cannot be re-sterilized.

Heterotopic bone and ankylosis can develop in the coronoid area, although uncommon, following coronoidectomy usually related to an inflammatory process or connective tissue/autoimmune disease, independent of the TMJ pathology (Fig. 9.5a, b). The bone usually develops along the path of the temporalis muscle tendon, even though the muscle may have been previously detached. It can develop in the presence of TMJ reconstruction with either autogenous tissue or TJP reconstruction. In some cases, the bone can extend posteriorly toward the joint. This coronoid-related heterotopic bone can cause pain, headaches, and decreased jaw function. It can usually be identified on CBCT, CT scans, or a panorex. The treatment protocol includes an intraoral approach to the coronoid

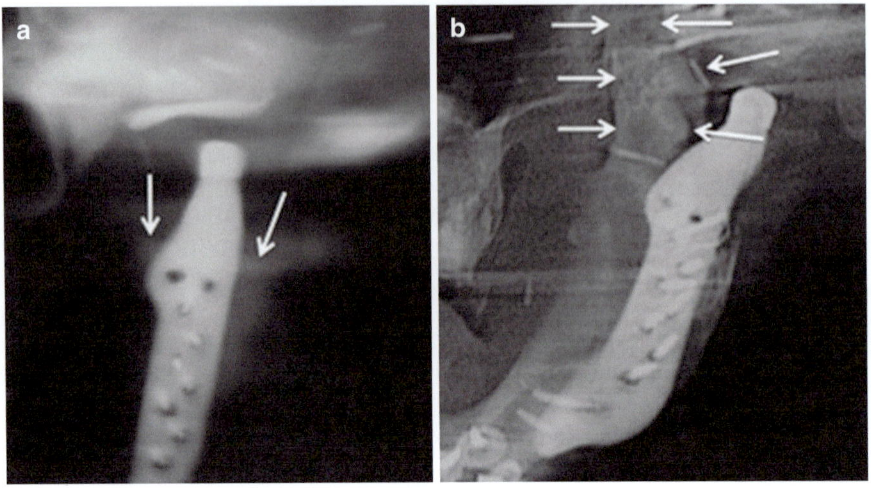

Fig. 9.5 (**a**, **b**) 36-year-old hemifacial microsomia male patient with three failed previous rib grafts to left TMJ, all resulting in re-ankylosis. (**a**) Immediate postsurgery left TMJ tomogram showing TMJ custom TJP, fat graft, and level of bone cut at ramus (*white arrows*). (**b**) Redevelopment of heterotopic bone at coronoid area 6 years postsurgery, causing pain and limited jaw movement (*white arrows*). No bone formation directly around mandibular condylar component where fat grafts were previously placed

area with a vertical incision at the anterior aspect of the ramus, identification and resection of the heterotopic bone, and placement of a fat graft. It remains imperative that the TJP not be exposed during this process.

9.6 Surgical Protocol for Managing TMJ Ankylosis

Two-stage surgery is the most common and more fail-safe approach for patient-fitted prostheses. This may not be necessary for stock prostheses, but the altered anatomy can make a stock joint very challenging or impossible to fit. Stage one surgery involves releasing the ankylosis on a stereolithographic model during planning, duplicating heterotopic and reactive bone removal at surgery, debridement of the joint, recontouring the fossa, and placement of an alloplastic spacer such as silastic or polymethyl methacrylate cement, with or without maxillomandibular fixation (surgeon's option). A CT scan of jaws in the final occlusion or corrected by virtual surgical planning is then completed to produce a 3-D stereolithic model to aid the construction of the TJP to be inserted at stage two surgery (Fig. 9.6a–d).

If orthognathic surgery to correct a dentofacial deformity is also planned, virtual surgical planning (VSP) can then be completed to place the mandible and maxilla into the final position prior to construction of a 3D stereolithic model. If VSP is not available, a stereolithic model can be prepared from the CT scan and the maxillo-mandibular complex repositioned and ramus modified to ensure a 20 mm gap

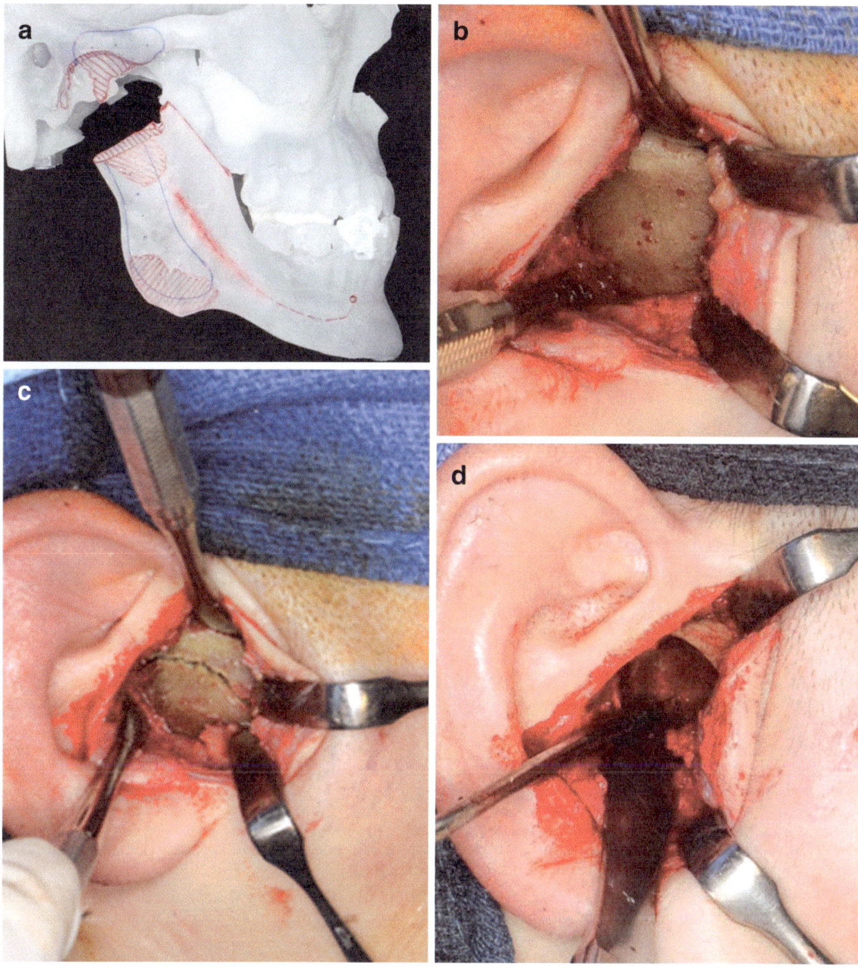

Fig. 9.6 (**a**) Presurgical model preparation with release of ankylosis, removal of condyle and heterotopic bone, joint debridement, creation of 20 mm space between fossa and ramus to accommodate the prosthesis. (**b**) Ankylosis of right TMJ with no clear delineation between condyle and fossa. (**c**) Bone cut through buccal cortex to define inferior rim of fossa. Heterotopic bone carefully removed. 20 mm vertical gap created between fossa and mandibular ramus to accommodate prosthesis. (**d**) Fossa debrided and recontoured to original bone level

between the glenoid fossa and the top of the ramus that is required to accommodate the TJP. The TJP can then be manufactured (Fig. 9.7a–c).

Stage-two surgery involves removing the spacer placed at stage one and debridement of the TMJ area. Contralateral mandibular ramus sagittal split osteotomy can be performed in an ipsilateral ankylosis requiring mandibular advancement followed by mobilizing of the mandible with counterclockwise rotation if indicated. Bilateral TMJ ankylosis will not require SSO as the mandible is advanced through the bilateral TJP but coronoidectomies will be necessary. The mandible is then

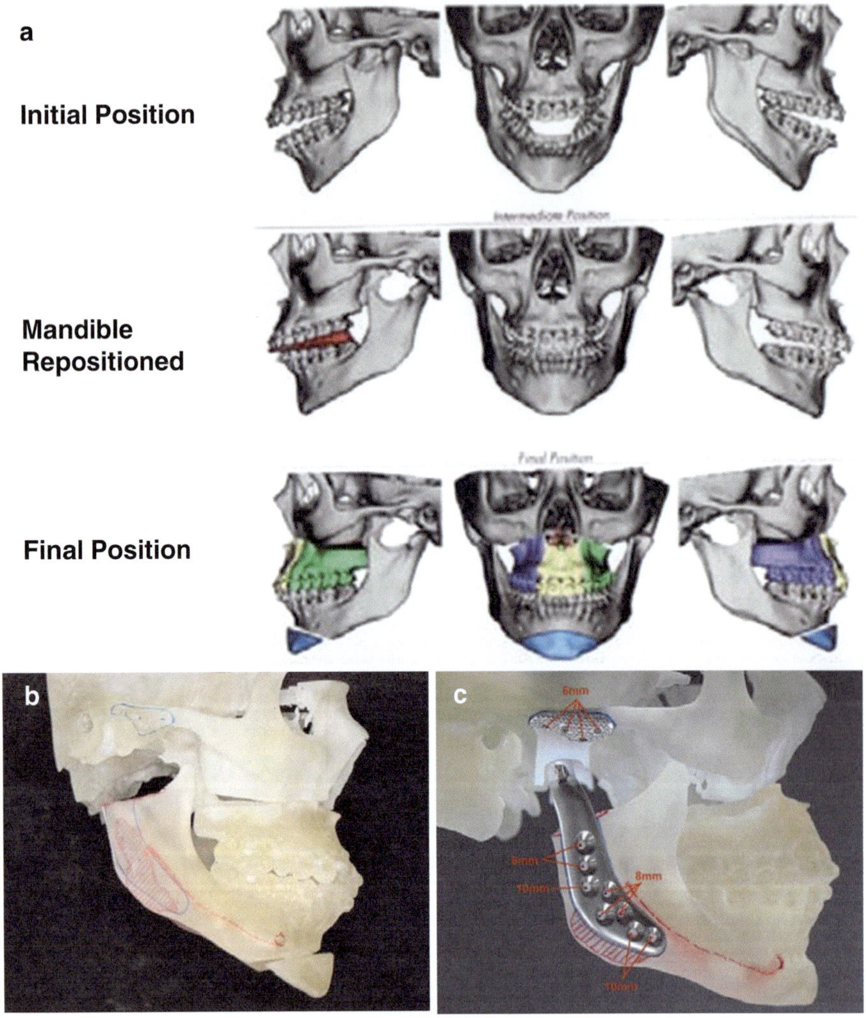

Fig. 9.7 (**a**) Virtual surgical planning (VSP) completed on the computer with the three primary stages printed out. (**b**) Stereolithic model printed with jaws in final position for presurgical preparation. (**c**) TMJ prosthesis manufactured on stereolithic model with suggested screw lengths listed

correctly positioned using the intermediate splint and intermaxillary fixation followed by implantation of the TMJ TJP and packing of fat graft around the articulating area of the prosthesis and closure of the TJP incisions (Figs. 9.4 and 9.6). In unilateral cases, the contralateral sagittal split osteotomy can then be fixated followed by performing the maxillary osteotomies if indicated. An advantage of two-stage surgery in ankylosis cases, particularly with decreased incisal opening that does not allow acquisition of dental impressions and models, is that after stage one, improvement in incisal opening may allow procurement of dental models to facilitate construction of surgical splints. For one-stage surgery, the splints can be constructed by the VSP company from the computer generated model but are not as accurate.

The technique for one-stage surgery requires substantial surgeon experience and skill to prevent unfavorable outcomes and complications. A CT scan of jaws and TMJs is completed prior to VSP to complete the ankylosis release and place the mandible in the final position. Conversely, a 3D stereolithic model can be made, and the surgeon can complete the ankylosis release and reposition the mandible manually. The custom-fitted prostheses can then be made. The challenge comes during the surgery in that the surgeon must accurately duplicate the planned surgery from the VSP or stereolithic model during the patient's procedure. Failure to complete this adequately may prevent the custom TJP from fitting. Concomitant orthognathic surgery can also be performed in one-stage surgery although again the surgeon's ability to complete the TMJ and orthognathic surgery depends on the ability to duplicate the planned ankylosis release and bone removal intraoperatively.

With the two-stage or one-stage surgery, if orthognathic surgery is also planned, VSP can greatly assist with positioning the mandible and maxilla in their final position [78–81]. Dental models are procured, dental model surgery performed, and models sent to the VSP Company for incorporation into the computer-simulated model. Obtaining dental models can be difficult or impossible to obtain due to the ankylosis which may influence the choice of one-stage versus two-stage surgery, the possibility for concomitant orthognathic surgery, or the ability to use intraoperative splints. In cases requiring double-jaw surgery with the total joint prostheses, it is usually easier to reposition the mandible to its final position first utilizing the intermediate splint and then placing the TMJ prostheses to stabilize the mandible in its new position, followed by repositioning the maxilla and then other ancillary procedures [80, 81].

9.7 Pediatric Considerations

In pediatric cases with bilateral TMJ ankylosis requiring double-jaw orthognathic surgery, females who are 13 years or older and males 15 years or older can be treated with the adult protocol as described above in a single surgical stage. This is because the total joint prostheses have no growth potential, and the maxilla will have no anteroposterior growth after the Le Fort I osteotomy, so the occlusion will remain stable although the subsequent facial growth vector will be downward and backward until cessation of the vertical alveolar bone growth [82–84]. Unilateral TMJ ankylosis can usually be treated in one surgical stage at age 15 years for females and 17–18 years for males with highly predictable results without potential adverse effects of normal jaw growth of the contralateral mandible. The above referenced ages for surgical intervention are guidelines established by the author, but there may be growth maturation differences for individual patients that require consideration and may alter the timing for surgical intervention. However, in TMJ ankylosis cases, early surgery may be indicated for functional, pain, or psychological reasons.

It has not been established as to how young a patient can be treated with a total joint prosthesis. However, in younger pediatric cases (ages 6 years or older), the treatment protocol can be separated into two stages. The first surgical stage includes release of the ankylosed TMJ, removal of the condyle, heterotopic and reactive bone, coronoidectomy if the ramus is to be significantly vertically lengthened or advanced, placement of TJP, fat graft and contralateral sagittal split, or inverted "L" osteotomy of the ramus if the mandible is being lengthened. In these younger patients, maxillary osteotomies are not recommended due to adverse effects on maxillary growth.

If surgery is performed at an early age, the patient should be followed until maxillofacial growth has been completed at approximately 15 years of age in females and 17–18 years of age in males [85, 86]. At this point, the residual dentofacial deformity and malocclusion can be reevaluated and corrected by maxillary and mandibular orthognathic surgery. For the second surgical stage, the case is treated as a typical dentofacial deformity case with a sagittal split osteotomy on the contralateral side if the patient was originally with a unilateral ankylosis, mandibular advancement, and maxillary surgery. The advancement of the mandible on the TMJ total joint prosthesis side can be accomplished by one of the four surgical options including extraoral sagittal split ramus osteotomy; intraoral ramus sagittal split osteotomy; advancing the mandible forward relative to the prosthesis by removing the screws from the mandibular component, advancing the mandible, and re-fixating the prosthesis with bone screws to the mandible in its new position; or replacing the mandibular component of the total joint prosthesis with a new longer mandibular component that would be reattached to the mandibular ramus after the mandible is moved into its new position.

Wolford and colleagues [21–33, 75, 76], Mercuri and colleagues [34–44], and others [45–47] have published numerous studies in reference to outcome data using TMJ Concepts patient-fitted TJP. A summary of these publications has produced the following facts in reference to these TJP: (1) TMJ Concepts patient-fitted TJP are superior to autogenous tissues for end-stage TMJ reconstruction relative to subjective and objective outcomes. (2) After two previous TMJ surgeries, autogenous tissues have a high failure rate, whereas patient-fitted total joint prostheses have a high success rate. (3) No donor site morbidity (except for the fat graft donor site). (4) Increased number of previous TMJ surgeries produces a lower level of improvement related to pain and function outcomes compared to patients with zero to one previous TMJ surgeries. (5) Failed TMJ alloplastic reconstruction (i.e., Proplast-Teflon, Silastic, metal-on-metal articulation) can create a foreign-body giant-cell reaction and/or metallosis, best treated by joint debridement and reconstruction with patient-fitted total joint prostheses. (6) Fat grafts packed around the articulating area of the prostheses improve outcomes relative to decreased pain, improved jaw function, and decreased requirement for repeat surgery. (7) Osseointegration of the TMJ Concepts fossa and mandibular components occurs and is important for long-term stability. (8) Posterior stop on the fossa component is important to stabilize the joint, jaw position, and occlusion. (9) Concomitant orthognathic surgery can be performed at the same time as the TMJs are reconstructed. (10) A 20-year follow-up study demonstrated improvements in pain, jaw function, diet, incisal opening, and quality of life as well as no requirements for prosthesis replacement due to wear or material failure [29].

For adult and most pediatric patients with TMJ heterotopic bone or ankylosis, with or without a coexisting dentofacial deformity, the most predictable method to address the TMJ pathology and jaw deformity includes TMJ reconstruction using patient-fitted TJP, fat grafts packed around the articulating area of the prostheses, and concomitant orthognathic surgery if indicated.

9.8 Case Presentation

A 15-year-old male presented with limited opening, jaw deformity, and difficulty in eating. The right TMJ ankylosis occurred before 4 years of age necessitating a rib graft at 6 years which re-ankylosed. Debridement of the right TMJ at 9 years was followed by re-ankylosis shortly after surgery. At age 15 years, he reported no TMJ pain, myofascial pain, or headaches. Jaw function was self-rated as poor. Examination showed he had a retruded maxilla and mandible, facial asymmetry with the mandible shifted significantly toward the right side. There was a transverse cant in the occlusal plane with the right side being elevated 4 mm compared to the left side. Maximal incisal opening was 12 mm. The patient's diagnoses included right TMJ ankylosis, left TMJ arthritis, and articular disc dislocation without reduction, maxillary anteroposterior and posterior vertical hypoplasia, mandibular anteroposterior and posterior vertical hypoplasia, occlusal cant, high occlusal plane angle, severely decreased oropharyngeal airway, Class I cuspid relationship on the right side, and Class II cuspid relationship on the left side (Fig. 9.8a–g).

The patient's treatment plan was as follows:

1. CT scans of jaws and jaw joints (Fig. 9.9a)
2. Cephalometric analysis and surgical treatment objectives (Fig. 9.9b, c)
3. One-stage surgery to:
   (a) Release of right TMJ/mandibular ankylosis with removal of heterotopic bone
   (b) Bilateral TMJ TJP reconstruction and mandibular advancement with counterclockwise rotation
   (c) Multiple maxillary osteotomies to advance in a counterclockwise direction
   (d) Left coronoidectomy

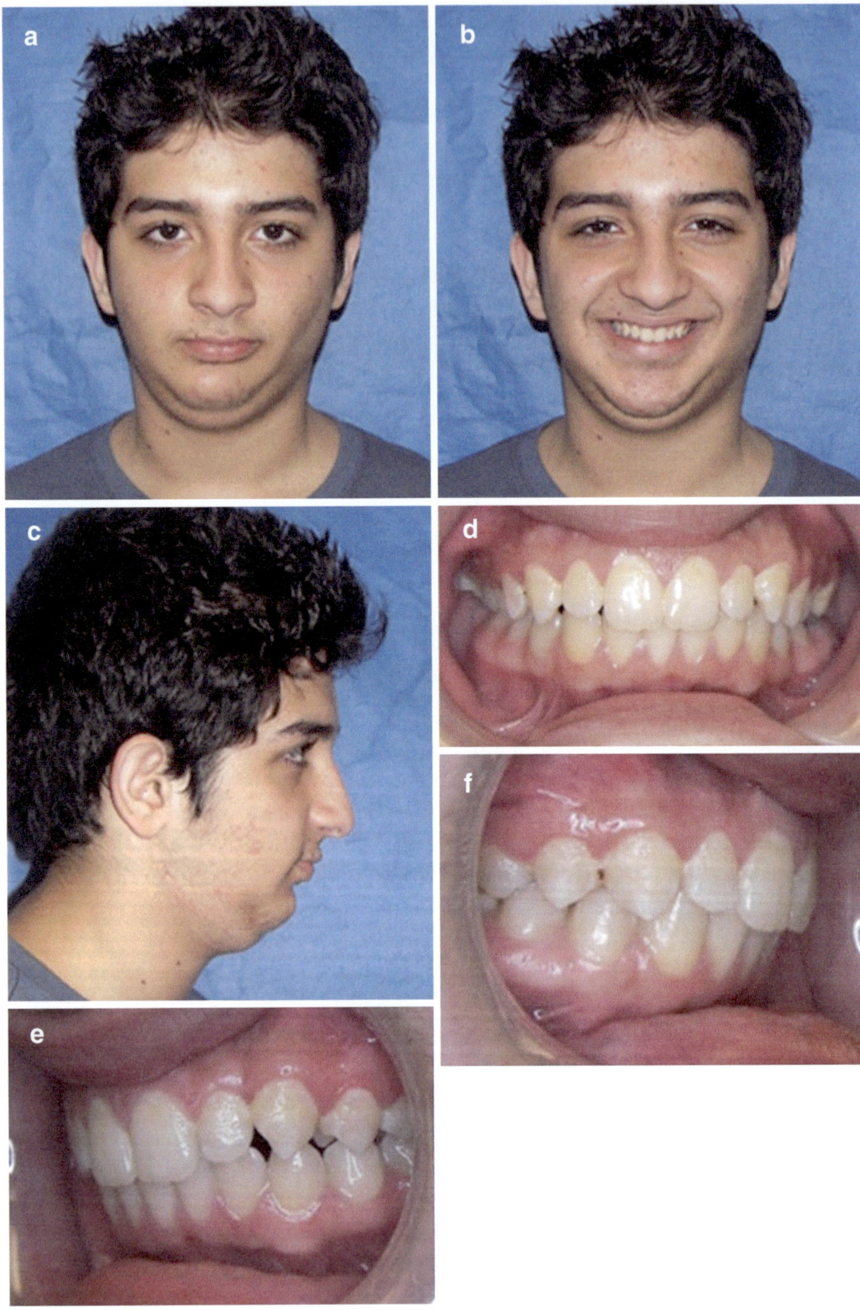

Fig. 9.8 15-year-old male with right TMJ ankylosis, retruded maxilla and mandible, facial asymmetry, and limited jaw function. (**a**) Frontal view, (**b**) frontal view smiling, (**c**) profile view, (**d–f**) occlusion

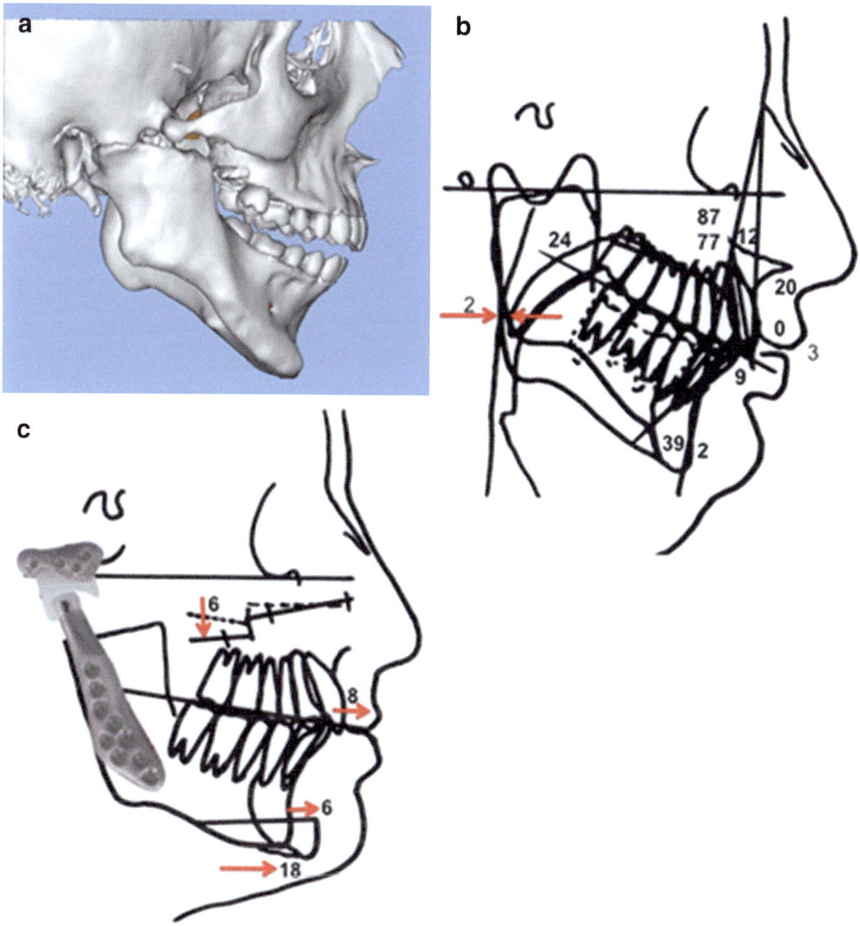

Fig. 9.9 (**a**) Presurgery 3D CT scan shows the ankylosed right TMJ. (**b**) Presurgical cephalometric analysis demonstrating retruded maxilla and mandible as well as the high occlusal plane angle facial morphology. (**c**) The surgical treatment objective demonstrates the counterclockwise rotation of the maxillomandibular complex and bony genioplasty with improved facial balance as the maxillary incisors advance 8 mm, pogonion advances 18 mm, and the occlusal plane decreases 16°

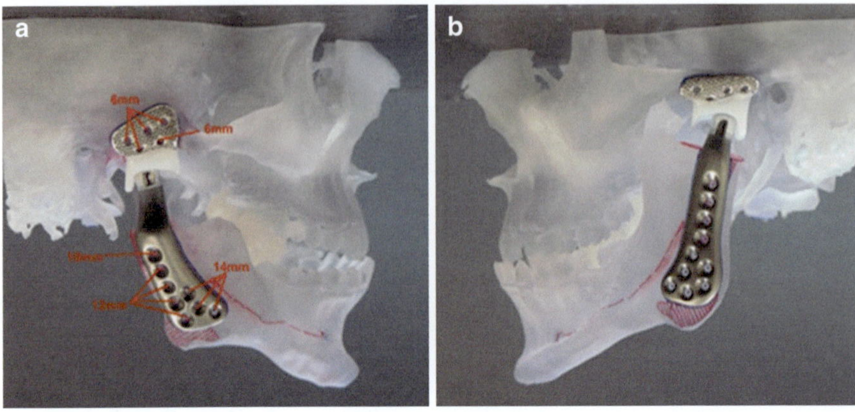

Fig. 9.10 (**a**, **b**) Photos of manufactured TMJ Concepts total joint prostheses on the stereolithic model for this case presentation, (**a**) right TMJ prosthesis, (**b**) left TMJ prosthesis

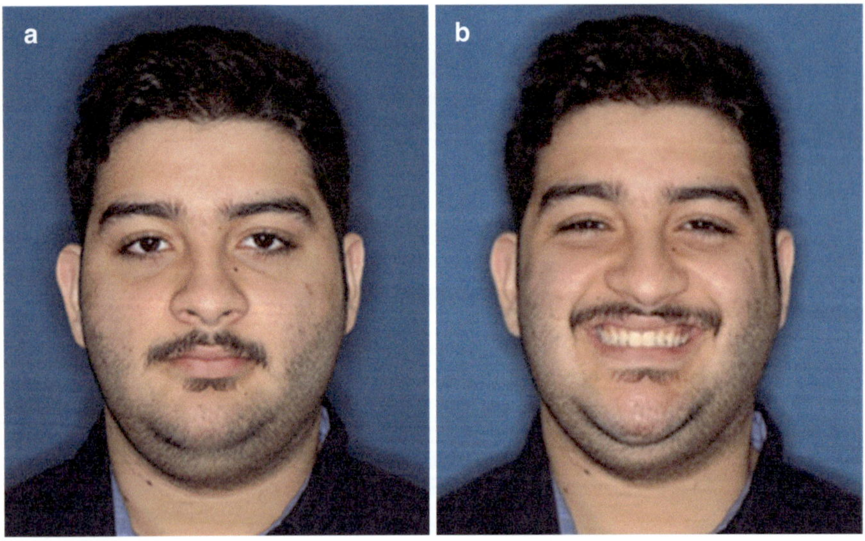

Fig. 9.11 (**a**–**f**) The patient is seen 5 years postsurgery with improved facial balance and function: (**a**) frontal view, (**b**) frontal view smiling, (**c**) profile view, (**d**–**f**) occlusion

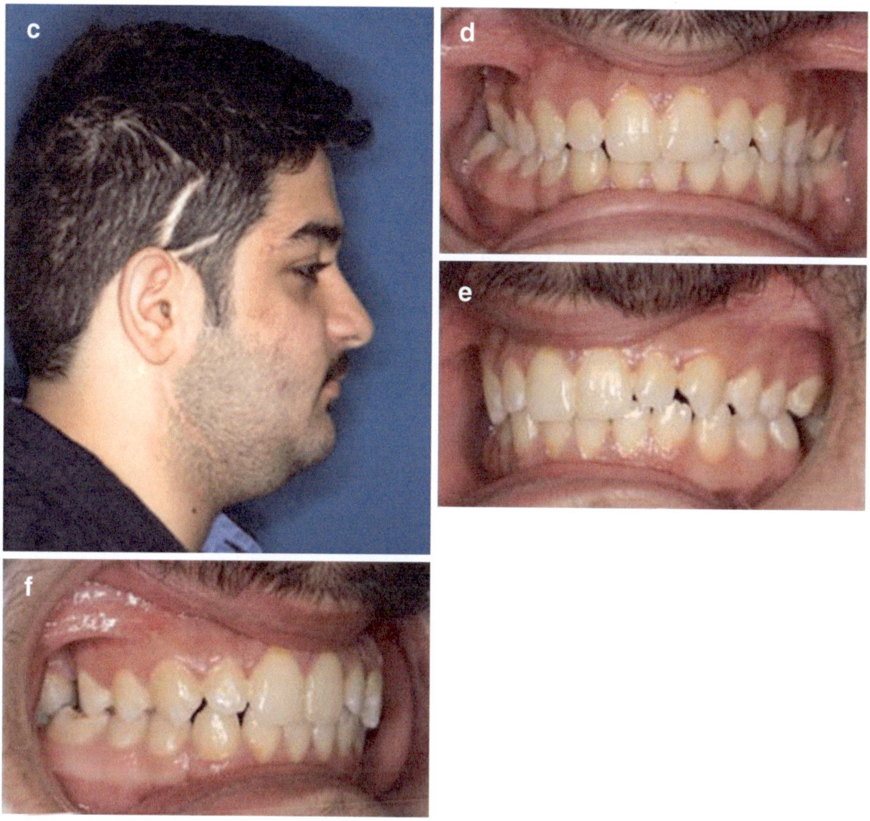

Fig. 9.11 (continued)

(e) Bilateral TMJ fat grafts packed around the articulating areas of the total joint prostheses
(f) Genioplasty (6 mm) (Fig. 9.10a, b)

Follow-up at 5 years revealed a stable result with good facial symmetry, no pain, and normal range of motion (Fig. 9.11a–f).

References

1. Hall BK. Cartilage. Biomedical aspects. New York: Academic Press; 1988. p. 322–3.
2. Wolford LM, Cassano DS, Goncalves JR. Common TMJ disorders: orthodontic and surgical management. In: McNamara JA, Kapila SD, editors. Temporomandibular disorders and orofacial pain: separating controversy from consensus, Craniofacial Growth Series, vol. 46. Ann Arbor (MI): The University of Michigan; 2009. p. 159–98.
3. Wolford LM, Movahed R. Concomitant TMJ and orthognathic surgery: diagnosis and treatment planning. Oral and maxillofacial surgery knowledge update. Chicago: AAOMS; 2014.

4. Wolford LM, Dhameja A. Planning for combined TMJ arthroplasty and orthognathic surgery. Ness GM (Guest Ed.). Atlas of the oral and maxillofacial clinics of North America. Philadelphia: WB Saunders Co.; 2011. p. 243–270.
5. Wolford LM. Mandibular asymmetry: temporomandibular joint degeneration. In: Bagheri SC, Bell RB, Khan HA, editors. Current therapy in oral and maxillofacial surgery. St. Louis: Elsevier Saunders; 2012. p. 696–725.
6. Wolford LM. Surgical planning in orthognathic surgery (chapter 60). In: Booth PW, Schendel SA, Hausamen JE, editors. Maxillofacial surgery volume 2. St Louis: Churchill Livingstone; 2007. p. 1155–210.
7. Wolford, LM, Stevo ELL, Alexander CM, Goncalves JR, Rodrigues DB. Orthodontics for orthognathic surgery. In Miloro M, Ghali GE, Larsen P, Waite P, editors. Peterson's principles of oral and maxillofacial surgery. Shelton: People's Medical Publishing House-USA; 2012, Chapter 55. p. 1263–1294.
8. Wolford LM, Fields RT Jr.. Diagnosis and treatment planning for orthognathic surgery. In: Betts N, Turvey T, editors. Volume 2, in Fonseca (Ed.) oral and maxillofacial surgery, Chapter 2. 2000. p. 24–55.
9. Wolford LM, Henry CH, Nikaein A, Newman JT, Namey TC. The temporomandibular joint alloplastic implant problem. In: Sessle BJ, Bryant PS, Dionne RA, editors. Temporomandibular disorders and related pain conditions. Seattle, WA: IASP Press; 1995. p. 443–7.
10. Wolford LM. Temporomandibular joint devices: treatment factors and outcomes. Oral Surg Oral Med Oral Pathol Oral Radiol Endod. 1997;83:143–9.
11. Matukas VJ, Szvmela VF, Schmidt JF. Surgical treatment of bony ankylosis in a child using a composite cartilage-bone iliac crest graft. J Oral Surg. 1980;38:903.
12. Dingman RO, Grabb WG. Reconstruction of both mandibular condyles with metatarsal bone grafts. Plast Reconstr Surg. 1964;34:441.
13. MacIntosh RB, Henny FA. A spectrum of application of autogenous costochondral grafts. J Maxillofac Surg. 1977;5257
14. Wolford LM, Cottrell DA, Henry CH. Sternoclavicular grafts for temporomandibular joint reconstruction. J Oral Maxillofac Surg. 1994;52:119–28.
15. Posnick JC, Goldstein JA. Surgical management of temporomandibular joint ankylosis in the pediatric population. Plast Reconstr Surg. 1993;91:791.
16. Pensler JM, Christopher RD, Bewyer DC. Correction of micrognathia with ankylosis of the temporomandibular joint in childhood. Plast Reconstr Surg. 1933;91:799.
17. Lindquist C, Pihakari A, Tasanen A, et al. Autogenous costochondral grafts in temporomandibular joint arthroplasty: a surgery of 66 arthroplasties in 60 patients. J Maxillofac Surg. 1986;14:143.
18. Munro IR, Chen YR, Park BY. Simultaneous total correction of temporomandibular ankylosis and facial asymmetry. Plast Reconstr Surg. 1986;77:517.
19. Perrot DH, Kaban LB. Temporomandibular joint ankylosis in children. Oral Maxillofac Surg Clin North Am. 1994;6:187.
20. Kaban LB, Perrot DH, Fisher K. A protocol for management of temporomandibular joint ankylosis. J Oral Maxillofac Surg. 1990;48:11.
21. Henry CH, Wolford LM. Treatment outcomes for temporomandibular joint reconstruction after Proplast Teflon implant failure. J Oral Maxillofac Surg. 1993;51:352.
22. Wolford LM, Cottrell DA, Henry CH. Temporomandibular joint reconstruction of the complex patient with the Techmedica custom-made total joint prosthesis. J Oral Maxillofac Surg. 1994;52:2–10.
23. Wolford LM, Pitta MC, Reiche-Fischel O, Franco PF. TMJ Concepts/Techmedica custom-made TMJ total joint prosthesis: 5-year follow-up study. Int J Oral Maxillofac Surg. 2003;32:268.
24. Wolford LM, Dingwerth DJ, Talwar RM, Pitta MC. Comparison of 2 temporomandibular joint total joint prosthesis systems. J Oral Maxillofac Surg. 2003;61:685–90.

25. Wolford LM, Pinto LP, Cardenas LE, Molina OR. Outcomes of treatment with custom-made temporomandibular joint total joint prostheses and maxillomandibular counter-clockwise rotation. Bayl Univ Med Cent Proc. 2008;21:18–24.
26. Coleta KED, Wolford LM, Goncalves JR, Santos-Pinto A, Pinto LP, Cassano DS. Maxillo-mandibular counter-clockwise rotation and mandibular advancement with TMJ concepts1 total joint prostheses: part I skeletal and dental stability. Int J Oral Maxillofac Surg. 2008;38:126–38.
27. Pinto LP, Wolford LM, Buschang PH, Bernardi FH, Goncalves JR, Cassano DS. Maxillo-mandibular counter-clockwise rotation and mandibular advancement with TMJ concepts total joint prostheses: part III pain and dysfunction outcomes. Int J Oral Maxillofac Surg. 2009;38:326–31.
28. Wolford LM, Bourland TC, Rodrigues D, Perez DE, Limoeiro E. Successful reconstruction of non-growing hemifacial microsomia patients with unilateral temporomandibular joint total joint prosthesis and orthognathic surgery. J Oral Maxillofac Surg. 2012;70:2835–53.
29. Wolford LM, Mercuri LG, Schneiderman ED, Movahed R, Allen W. Twenty-year follow-up study on a patient-fitted temporomandibular joint prosthesis: the techmedica/TMJ concepts device. J Oral Maxillofac Surg. 2015;73:952–60.
30. Perez D, Wolford LM, Schneiderman E, Movahed R, Bourland C, Perez E. Does unilateral temporomandibular total joint reconstruction result in contralateral joint pain and dysfunction? J Oral Maxillofac Surg. 2016;74(8):1539–47. doi:10.1016/j.joms.2016.02.009.
31. Wolford L, Movahed R, Teschke M, Fimmers R, Havard D, Schneiderman E. Temporomandibular joint ankylosis can be successfully treated with TMJ concepts patient-fitted total joint prosthesis and autogenous fat grafts v12-21-15. J Oral Maxillofac Surg. 2016;74(6):1215–27. doi:10.1016/j.joms.2016.01.017.
32. Wolford LM, Movahed R. Combined TMJ and orthognathic surgery. In: Kademani D, Tiwana P, editors. Atlas of oral and maxillofacial surgery: Elsevier Saunders; 2016. p. 1364–77.
33. Wolford LM. Concomitant TMJ total joint replacement and orthognathic surgery. In: Mercuri LG, editor. Temporomandibular Joint Total Joint Replacement – TMJ TJR. Switzerland: Springer International Publishing; 2016. p. 133–64.
34. Mercuri LG, Wolford LM, Sanders B, White RD, Hurder A, Henderson W. Custom CAD/CAM total temporomandibular joint reconstruction system: preliminary multicenter report. J Oral Maxillofac Surg. 1995;53:106–15.
35. Mercuri LG. Alloplastic temporomandibular joint reconstruction. Oral Surg Oral Med Oral Pathol. 1998;85:631.
36. Mercuri LG. Subjective and objective outcomes for patients reconstructed with a patient-fitted total temporomandibular joint prosthesis. J Oral Maxillofac Surg. 1999;57:1427–30.
37. Mercuri LG. The TMJ concepts patient fitted total temporomandibular joint reconstruction prosthesis. Oral Maxillofac Surg Clin North Am. 2000;12:73
38. Mercuri LG. The use of alloplastic prostheses for temporomandibular joint reconstruction. J Oral Maxillofac Surg. 2000;58:70.
39. Mercuri LG. The TMJ concepts patient-fitted total temporomandibular joint reconstruction prosthesis. Oral Maxillofac Surg Clin North Am. 2000;12:73.
40. Mercuri LG, Wolford LM, Sanders B, White RD, Giobbie-Hurder A. Long-term follow-up of the CAD/CAM patient fitted total temporomandibular joint reconstruction system. J Oral Maxillofac Surg. 2002;60:1440–8.
41. Mercuri LG, Giobbi-Hurder A. Long term outcomes after total alloplastic TMJ reconstruction following exposure to failed materials. J Oral Maxillofac Surg. 2004;62:1088–96.
42. Mercuri LG, Edibam NR, Giobbie-Hurder A. Fourteen-year follow-up of a patient-fitted total temporomandibular joint reconstruction system. J Oral Maxillofac Surg. 2007;65:1140–8.
43. Mercuri LG. Temporomandibular joint reconstruction. In: Fonseca R, editor. Oral and maxillofacial surgery. Philadelphia: Elsevier ; 2008. p. 945–60.Chapter 51
44. Mercuri LG. End-stage TMD and TMJ reconstruction. In: Miloro M, Ghali G, Larsen P, Waite P, editors. Peterson's principles of oral & maxillofacial surgery. 3rd ed. PMPH, USA Ltd; 2012. Chapter 52. p. 1173–1186.

45. Mehra P, Wolford LM, Baran S, Cassano DS. Single-stage comprehensive surgical treatment of the rheumatoid arthritis temporomandibular joint patient. J Oral Maxillofac Surg. 2009;67:1859–72.
46. Sidebottom AJ, Gruber E. One-year prospective outcome analysis and complications following total replacement of the TMJ with the TMJ Concepts System. Br J Oral Maxillofac Surg. 2013;51:620–4.
47. Murdock B, Buchanan J, Cliff J. TMJ replacement: a New Zealand perspective. Int J Oral Maxillofac Surg. 2014;43:595–9.
48. Wolford LM, Karras SC. Autologous fat transplantation around temporomandibular joint total joint prostheses: preliminary treatment outcomes. J Oral Maxillofac Surg. 1997;55:245–51.
49. Francis MD, Russell RCG, Fleisch H. Diphosphonates inhibit formation of calcium phosphate crystals in vitro and pathologic calcification in vivo. Science. 1969;165:1264–6.
50. Ritter MA, Gioe TJ. The effect of indomethacin on para-articular ectopic ossification following total hip arthroplasty. Clin Orthop. 1982;167:113–7.
51. Durr ED, Turlington EG, Foote RL. Radiation treatment of heterotopic bone formation in the temporomandibular joint articulation. Int J Radiat Oncol Biol Phys. 1993;27:863–9.
52. Jensen AW, Viozzi CF, Foote RL. Long-term results of radiation prophylaxis for heterotopic ossification in the temporomandibular joint. J Oral Maxillofac Surg. 2010;68:1100–5.
53. Roychoudhury A, Parkash H, Trikha A. Functional restoration by gap arthroplasty in temporomandibular joint ankylosis: a report of 50 cases. Oral Surg Oral Med Oral Pathol Oral Radiol Endod. 1999;87:166–9.
54. Erol B, Tanrikulu R, Görgün B. A clinical study on ankylosis of the temporomandibular joint. J Craniomaxillofac Surg. 2006;34:100–6.
55. Topazian RG. Comparision of the gap and interposition arthroplasty in treatment of temporomandibular ankylosis. J Oral Surg. 1966;24:405–9.
56. Yazdani J, Ali Ghavimi M, Pourshahidi S, Ebrahimi H. Comparison of clinical efficacy of temporalis myofascial flap and dermal graft as interpositional material in treatment of temporomandibular joint ankylosis. J Craniofac Surg. 2010;21:1218–20.
57. Mehrotra D, Pradhan R, Mohammad S, Jaiswara C. Random control trial of dermis-fat graft and interposition of temporalis fascia in the management of temporomandibular ankylosis in children. Br J Oral Maxillofac Surg. 2008;46(7):521–6.
58. Dimitroulis G. The interpositional dermis-fat graft in the management of temporomandibular joint ankylosis. Int J Oral Maxillofac Surg. 2004;33:755–60.
59. Dimitroulis G, Trost N, Morrison W. The radiological fate of dermis-fat grafts in the human temporomandibular joint using magnetic resonance imaging. Int J Oral Maxillofac Surg. 2008;37:249–54.
60. Kaban LB, Perrott DH, Fisher K. A protocol for management of temporomandibular joint ankylosis. J Oral Maxillofac Surg. 1990;48:1145–51.
61. Kaban LB, Bouchard C, Troulis MJ. A protocol for management of temporomandibular joint ankylosis in children. J Oral Maxillofac Surg. 2009;67(9):1966–78.
62. Balaji SM. Modified temporalis anchorage in craniomandibular reankylosis. Int J Oral Maxillofac Surg. 2003;32(5):480–5.61.
63. Blair VP. Operative treatment of ankylosis of the mandible. Trans South Surg Assoc. 1913;28:435.
64. Murphy JB. Arthroplasty for intra-articular bony and fibrous ankylosis of the temporomandibular articulation. JAMA. 1914;62:1783.
65. Merikanto JE, Alhopuro S, Ritsila VA. Free fat transplant prevents osseous reunion of skull defects. A new approach in the treatment of craniosynostosis. Scand J Plast Reconstr Surg. 1987;21:183–8.
66. Saunders MC, Keller JT, Dunsker SB, Mayfield FH. Survival of autogenous fat grafts in humans and in mice. Connect Tissue Res. 1981;8:85–91.
67. Yamaguchi M, Matsumoto F, Bujo H, Skibasaki M, Takahashi K, Yashimoto S, Kchinose M, Saito Y. Revascularization determines volume retention and gene expression by fat grafts in mice. Exp Biol Med. 2005;230:742–8.

68. Trevor PB, Martin RA, Saunders GK, Trotter EJ. Healing characteristics of free and pedicle fat grafts after dorsal laminectomy and duratomy in dogs. Vet Surg. 1991;20:282–90.
69. Qi Z, Li E, Wang H. Experimental study on free grafting of fat particles. Zhonghua Zheng Xing Shao Shang Wai Ke Za Zhi. 1997;13:54–6.
70. Wolford LM, Morales-Ryan CA, Garcia-Morales P, Cassano DS. Autologous fat grafts placed around Temporomandibular Joint (TMJ) total joint prostheses to prevent heterotopic bone. Bayl Univ Med Cent Proc. 2008;21:248–54.
71. Wolford LM, Cassano DS. Autologous fat grafts around Temporomandibular Joint (TMJ) total joint prostheses to prevent heterotopic bone. In: Shiffman MA, editor. Autologous fat transfer. Berlin/Heidelberg: Springer; 2010. p. 361–82.
72. Mercuri LG, Ali FA, Woolson R. Outcomes of total alloplastic replacement with periarticular autogenous fat grafting for management of reankylosis of the temporomandibular joint. J Oral Maxillofac Surg. 2008;66:1794–803.
73. Carpaneda CA, Ribeiro MT. Study of the histologic alterations and viability of the adipose graft in humans. Aesthetic Plast Surg. 1993;17:43–7.
74. Horl HW, Feller AM, Biemer E. Technique for liposuction fat reimplantation and long-term volume evaluation by magnetic resonance imaging. Ann Plast Surg. 1991;26:248–58.
75. Wolford LM, McPhillips A, Rodrigues D. TMJ ankylosis in children: comparison of 3 methods of joint reconstruction. AAOMS. 2009.
76. Frietas RZ, Mehra P, Wolford LM. Autogenous versus alloplastic TMJ reconstruction in rheumatoid-induced TMJ disease. J Oral Maxillofac Surg. 2002;58:43.
77. Saeed N, Hensher R, McLeod N, Kent J. Reconstruction of the TMJ Autogenous compared with Alloplastic. Br J Oral Maxillofac Surg. 2002;40:296–9.
78. Xia J, Ip HH, Samman N, et al. Computer-assisted three-dimensional surgical planning and simulation: 3D virtual osteotomy. Int J Oral Maxillofac Surg. 2000;29:11.
79. Gateno J, Xia J, Teichgraeber J, et al. Clinical feasibility of Computer-Aided Surgical Simulation (CASS) in the treatment of complex cranio-maxillofacial deformities. J Oral Maxillofac Surg. 2007;65:728.
80. Movahed R, Teschke M, Wolford LM. Protocol for concomitant temporomandibular joint custom-fitted total joint reconstruction and orthognathic surgery utilizing computer-assisted surgical simulation. J Oral Maxillofac Surg. 2013;71:2123–9.
81. Movahed R, Wolford LM. Protocol for concomitant temporomandibular joint custom-fitted total joint reconstruction and orthognathic surgery using computer-assisted surgical simulation. Oral Maxillofac Surg Clin N Am. 2015;27:37–45.
82. Wolford LM, Karras SC, Mehra P. Considerations for orthognathic surgery during growth, part 1: mandibular deformities. Am J Orthod Dentofacial Orthop. 2001;119:95–101.
83. Wolford LM, Karras SC, Mehra P. Considerations for orthognathic surgery during growth, part 2: maxillary deformities. Am J Orthod Dentofacial Orthop. 2001;119:102–5.
84. Wolford LM, Rodrigues DB. Orthognathic considerations in the young patient and effects on facial growth. In: Preedy VR, editor. Handbook of growth and growth monitoring in health and disease. New York: Springer; 2012. p. 1789–808.
85. Riolo ML, Moyers RE, McNamara JA, Hunter WS. An atlas of craniofacial growth: cephalometric standards from the University School Growth Study, The University of Michigan. Ann Arbor, MI: University of Michigan; 1974. p. 105–6.
86. Wolford LM, Rodrigues DB. Temporomandibular Joint (TMJ) pathologies in growing patients: effects on facial growth and development. In: Preedy VR, editor. Handbook of growth and growth monitoring in health and disease. New York: Springer; 2012. p. 1809–28.

Infection Following Total Joint Replacement

10

Louis G. Mercuri

10.1 Introduction

Ever since orthopedic total joint replacement (TJR) was introduced by Sir John Charnley [1], orthopedic joint replacement has gained popularity given the considerable improvement in biocompatibility, functionality, and durability of these devices [2, 3]. Many of these alloplastic joints can function properly for decades [4–6]. However, one of the potential drawbacks to this technological and clinical advancement in the management of end-stage joint disease is the susceptibility of these devices to infection. Management of these infections involves elimination of the infection and returning the joint to function. In order to achieve these goals, early diagnosis and a rational management plan that includes surgical intervention, combined with appropriate antibiotic therapy, are essential [7, 8].

The Medicare 5% national sample administrative database documents a 1.63% and 1.55% risk of infection within the first 2 years following primary total hip (THA) and knee arthroplasty (TKA), with an additional risk between 2 and 10 years of 0.59% and 0.46%, respectively [9, 10]. Further studies have suggested that both the incidence and prevalence of periprosthetic joint infection (PJI) is increasing with time, with the overall infection burden expected to rise to >6% in the coming years [11].

In a retrospective survey of 2476 TMJ TJR cases involving 3368 joints, there were 51 (1.51%) reported cases of infection in the postoperative period which ranged from 2 weeks to 12 years [12]. Despite these statistics that demonstrate postoperative TMJ TJR infection as relatively uncommon, the clinical, psychological,

L.G. Mercuri, DDS, MS
Department of Orthopedic Surgery, Rush University Medical Center, Chicago, IL, USA

TMJ Concepts, Ventura, CA, USA
e-mail: lgm@tmjconcepts.com

G.F. Bouloux (ed.), *Complications of Temporomandibular Joint Surgery*,
DOI 10.1007/978-3-319-51241-9_10

and economic consequences of this complication can be substantial. Therefore, the development of management algorithms based on early diagnostic testing has been the subject of continued exploration in the literature [13].

10.2 Pathophysiology

Prosthetic joint infections present characteristic signs that can be divided into acute manifestations (severe pain, high fever, toxemia, heat, rubor, and surgical wound discharges) and chronic manifestations without fever (progressive pain, skin fistulae, and drainage of purulent secretions). The clinical presentation depends on the virulence of the etiological organism, the nature of the infected tissue, the infection acquisition route, and the duration of disease evolution [14]. Early and delayed infections are both thought to be due to organisms introduced at the time of surgery, whereas late infections are more likely to have a hematogenous etiology [7]. Infecting organisms can form microcolonies on the prosthesis surfaces. These elaborate exopolysaccharides coalesce forming a biofilm. Once formed, organisms within the biofilm are protected from host immune responses and may display reduced susceptibility to antibiotics as a result of changes in metabolic processes and poor diffusion [15].

10.3 Prevention

The preoperative patient assessment remains paramount in being able to risk stratify patients contemplating TMJ TJR [16]. There are a number of endogenous (patient-related) and exogenous (process-/procedure-related) variables that affect a patient's risk for development of a surgically related infection. Some endogenous factors cannot be changed, such as age, gender, and genetic factors [17]. However, a number of exogenous factors may exist that can be improved to decrease the potential for the development of an infection [18]. Preoperative variables can be addressed to reduce the risk of complications.

10.3.1 Preoperative Considerations

10.3.1.1 Nutrition

TMJ TJR surgical candidates, such as those with ankylosis or other pathologic conditions that prevent them from maintaining a proper diet over an extended period of time, may require nutritional and hematologic evaluation and intervention before TMJ TJR. Possible interventions include family support discussions, diet counseling, vitamin and iron supplements, transfusion, and social service referrals. Depending on the surgical urgency, delay of surgery until the patient's nutritional and hematologic status improves may be indicated [19].

10.3.1.2 Systemic Disease Control

As with the implantation of any device into medically compromised patients, it is essential that any risk-related systemic pathology be under control before surgery. Conditions affecting the immune system including diabetes should be optimized prior to any surgery. Any dosage and/or medication modifications should be made in consultation with the patient's physician.

10.3.1.3 Smoking

Cigarette smoking is associated with inhibited wound healing and decreased circulation to the skin due to microvascular obstruction from platelet aggregation and increased nonfunctioning hemoglobin. In addition, smoking has been found to compromise the immune system and the respiratory system [20]. Smoking should be discontinued 6–8 weeks before surgery. In a randomized study, participation in a preoperative smoking cessation program was found to reduce postoperative complication rates. No wound-related complications occurred in the patients who stopped smoking before surgery [21, 22]. Furthermore, in an experimental study, the use of transdermal nicotine patches during smoking cessation did not impair wound healing [23].

10.3.1.4 Preexisting Remote Site Infections

Infections at a site remote from the TJR have been linked to a three- to fivefold increase in surgical site infection rates [24]. The most common sources of blood-borne infection are the skin, urinary, and respiratory tracts. Therefore, any remote infections should be identified and managed before TMJ TJR. It is not uncommon for multiple dental extractions to be required in order for oral infections to be eliminated preoperatively. Although the underlying evidence is weak, it is advisable to perform dental extractions before TMJ TJR [25].

There are several operative variables that are thought to influence the risk of TJR infection that are amenable to intervention by the surgeon and operative team.

10.3.2 Perioperative Considerations

10.3.2.1 Skin

A Cochrane Database Review provided no clear evidence of benefit of preoperative showering or bathing with chlorhexidine over other wash products to reduce surgical infections. However, a benefit of day-of-surgery showering or bathing in an effort to reduce the incidence of nosocomial infections was demonstrated [26].

10.3.2.2 Pre-incision Antibiotic Prophylaxis

Systemic intravenous antibiotic prophylaxis reduces the risk of postoperative infection. Cephalosporins are widely used, based on their good efficacy against staphylococcal species and uropathogens. Vancomycin is indicated in high-risk patients carrying methicillin-resistant *Staphylococcus aureus* (MRSA). If the patient has an allergy to β-lactam antibiotics, clindamycin or vancomycin can be used [27]. Rosenberg [28] and Levant [29] demonstrated the importance of the administration of antibiotic prophylaxis 1 h before initiation of the skin incision in orthopedic joint replacement. Therefore, it is recommended that antibiotic administration be part of the "time-out" protocol to ensure compliance with the proper timing of prophylactic antibiotic administration in TMJ TJR cases.

10.3.2.3 Anesthesia

Contamination of the surgical site and/or displacement of the anesthetic naso-endotracheal tube (NET) during TMJ TJR can be avoided by suturing the NET to the nasal septum. The NET, as well as associated tubing and equipment, can then be directed caudally and away from the surgical field decreasing the potential for NET contamination of the sterile field and/or its displacement [30].

10.3.2.4 Eyes

After the patient is anesthetized and the airway is secured, the eyes should be lubricated, taped shut, and protected to prevent corneal injury, conjunctivitis from blood/irrigation, or contamination of the surgical field [30].

10.3.2.5 Hair

After shearing, not shaving, the hair to above the ear, the remaining hair should be drawn up toward the crown of the head, away from the planned incision sites. Foam tape can be used to wrap the head circumferentially (forehead–above the ear–occiput) so that the hair will be kept out of the surgical field [30].

10.3.2.6 Ear

Thorough irrigation of the auditory canal with a gentle bactericidal solution should be performed before skin preparation and final sterile draping. The external auditory canal should be occluded to prevent wound contamination during surgery from the egress of bacterial flora and/or accumulation of irrigation fluid and/or blood intra-operatively. A cotton pledget moistened with sterile mineral oil provides one among many occlusive options [30].

10.3.2.7 Oral Cavity

Any intraoral procedures such as application of maxillomandibular fixation (arch bars, Oliver Loops, fixation screws, etc.) should be completed before skin preparation and final sterile draping. All contaminated intraoral instruments and power equipment must remain separate from the sterile instruments to be used in the sterile surgical field. After appropriate skin preparation, in unilateral cases, a plastic-adhesive isolation drape (e.g., 1010 Steri-drape®[1]) should be used from the contralateral submental area to the ipsilateral temporal area to isolate the mouth from the sterile surgical field. This type of draping allows access to the oral cavity while maintaining sterility at the surgical sites [30]. In bilateral TMJ TJR cases, to avoid

[1] ®3 M Health Care, St Paul, MN.

contamination when turning the head, the mouth should be sealed with a plastic-adhesive occlusive dressing (Tegaderm Film®[2] or Opsite®[3]). The sutured NET and the nose can be further isolated using the bilateral 1010 Steri-drapes, as described above, folding the loose ends together over the NET and the nose in a sterile fashion. The loose ends should be sealed together using Steri-Strips®[4] [30].

10.3.2.8 Pre-incision Skin Preparation

This is of critical importance, ensuring not only that the antibacterial solution used has broad-spectrum properties but also that the product is properly applied to avoid oral contamination of the surgical incision sites. Additional strategies used to reduce bacterial migration into the surgical incision include the use of antiseptic impregnated adhesive drapes and/or novel cyanoacrylate-based skin sealants that can be applied over the skin preparation site to immobilize residual skin flora, including those imbedded in hair follicles [31].

10.3.3 Intraoperative Considerations

10.3.3.1 Incisions

The incisions for access to the surgical site must be large enough to expeditiously execute the procedure. Small incisions, though potentially less conspicuous, may require more forceful retraction, requiring excessive traction on the wound skin edges, resulting in ischemia. This can lead to poor healing, increasing the potential for infection, or excessive scarring. Precise wound closure is an important to assure proper healing, thereby decreasing the incidence of infection [30].

10.3.3.2 Parotid Gland

Parotid gland tissue is typically encountered during TMJ TJR surgery. Care should be observed during dissection, retraction, instrumentation, and use of power equipment to avoid injury to parotid tissue. Injury to this tissue can result in the contamination of the surrounding host bone, tissue, and device components with potentially bacteria laden saliva [30].

10.3.3.3 TMJ TJR Components

Direct contamination of the devices before implantation from improper handling in the operating room environment or indirect contamination from the skin, ear flora, or saliva during multiple "try ins" of templates and/or device components can result in infection. Mercuri and Psutka state that it appears prudent to soak the components and then copiously irrigate the surgical access wounds with antibiotic or antibacterial solution before closure [12].

---

[2] ®3 M Health Care, St. Paul, MN.

[3] ®Smith & Nephew, London, England.

[4] ®3 M Health Care, St. Paul, MN.

10.3.3.4 Hemostasis, Irrigation and Drains

Intraoperatively and before wound closure, the surgeon must ensure that adequate hemostasis has been achieved to prevent the formation of a hematoma. Hematomas have been implicated not only in the development of infections [32] but also in the need for revision surgery after TJR [33]. Copious irrigation with saline or antibiotic solution to remove any clotted blood, soft tissue, and bony fragments before wound closure is extremely important in decreasing the potential for a postoperative infection. The author considers the use of drains as a potential source of contamination and prefers meticulous attention to hemostasis to the use of either active or passive drains [30].

10.3.4 Postoperative Considerations

10.3.4.1 Auditory Canal

After precise and careful wound closure, an ear speculum should be used to inspect the auditory canal and tympanic membrane to ensure that there was no intraoperative accumulation of irrigation fluid, blood, or iatrogenic perforations unintentionally created in the auditory canal or the tympanic membrane. The results of this inspection should be documented in the operative notes. Blood clots should be removed with gentle, warm saline irrigation and careful suction. Instillation of antibiotic/steroid otic drops and occlusion of the external auditory meatus with a cotton pledget is recommended to decrease the potential for the development of infection and/or inflammation of the auditory canal and/or tympanic membrane. If a perforation of the auditory canal or tympanic membrane is discovered during this examination, consultation with an otolaryngologist is advised to determine the best management options [30].

10.3.4.2 Pressure Dressing

A pressure dressing should be applied for a minimum of 8–12 h to aid in minor hemostasis and assist in the reduction of edema.

10.3.4.3 Postimplantation Antibiotics

There appears to be little consensus on the need for postimplantation antibiotics in orthopedic TJR [34]. Until similar studies are available for TMJ TJR, an antibiotic that covers the spectrum of potential skin, ear, and saliva contaminants (i.e., clindamycin and cephradine) is recommended for 7–10 days postoperatively, especially for the high-risk patient [12].

10.3.4.4 Nosocomial Infections

Although nosocomial infections are difficult to predict and manage, the duration of hospitalization should be minimized to reduce the risk of colonization of the patient's skin with hospital-acquired organisms. Meticulous wound care and personal hygiene (hand washing) by both the surgeon and patient both during hospitalization and after discharge are absolutely essential [30].

10.3.5 Discharge Considerations and Information

The risk of infection continues even after the patient leaves the hospital. Surgeons should educate patients and their relatives regarding proper wound care, personal hygiene, how to recognize early signs of an impending infection, and the importance of reporting symptoms to their surgeons as soon as any arise. Providing preprinted instructional information and answers to frequently asked questions should be considered [30].

10.4 Postoperative Infection

10.4.1 Diagnosis

To date there is no test that produces "absolute" accuracy in the diagnosis of a periprosthetic joint infection (PJI) after joint replacement. Therefore, due to this lack of such a "gold standard," diverse and sometimes conflicting criteria have been proposed [13]. Based on the review of the TMJ TJR infection literature [12, 13, 29, 35] and the American Academy of Orthopedic Surgeons' (AAOS) Clinical Practice Guideline for Diagnosis of Periprosthetic Joint Infections [36], practical diagnostic and management algorithms were developed for early and delayed TMJ TJR infections.

10.4.1.1 Early TMJ TJR PJI

As with any diagnosis, the clinical history and physical examination are important. A suspected PJI occurring within days or <3 weeks after TMJ TJR typically manifests as increasing pain, low grade fever, swelling, and erythema at the preauricular and/or retromandibular incisions, as well as drainage from either or both surgical sites [35]. Erythrocyte sedimentation rate (ESR) and C-reactive protein (CRP) serology will be elevated as will the peripheral white blood cell count (WBC). There is no need to aspirate the joint, but if aspiration wound cultures are taken, they should be obtained before antibiotics are employed in order to assure proper identification of the etiologic organisms. (Fig. 10.1)

In early PJI cases, CT imaging will typically reveal a fluid collection and stable component fixation. Should there be any evidence of component or fixation loosening, these issues must be addressed along with the PJI to ensure resolution. Magnetic resonance imaging, ultrasound, and nuclear medicine scans are unnecessary in the diagnosis of an early TMJ TJR infection [35]. Wolford et al. discuss the management of early TMJ TJR infections [35]. The initial recommendation is that via the preauricular incision, the surface of the mandibular condyle and fossa component of the prostheses be thoroughly scrubbed with iodine solution using a sterile toothbrush. Next, irrigating catheters are placed through separate stab incisions above the preauricular incision and secured with sutures. One is placed on the lateral side of the mandibular component and ramus. The second is placed on the medial side of the articulating portion of the prosthesis. A Penrose drain is inserted through the retromandibular incision and positioned on the lateral aspect of the mandibular component

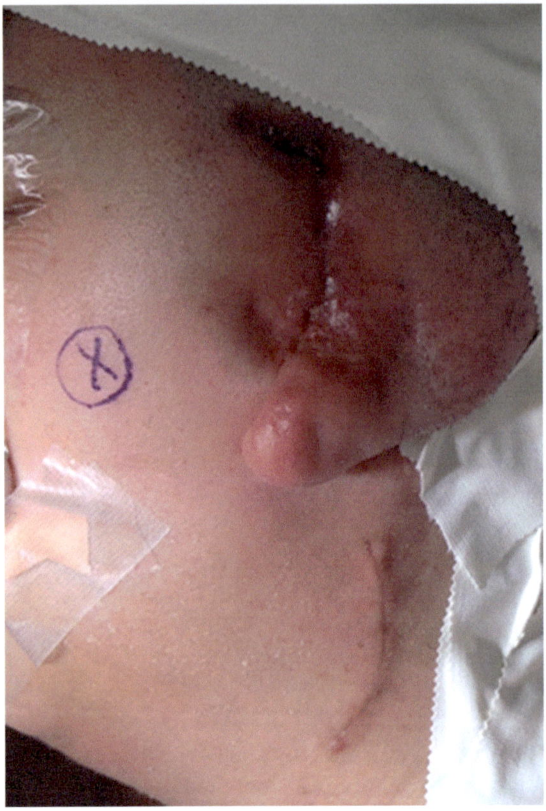

Fig. 10.1 Left TJR in a patient with hemifacial microsomia. Erythema, fluctuance, and suppuration with preauricular wound breakdown at 2 weeks postoperatively

Table 10.1 Algorithm for the management of an early TMJ TJR infection

	Early Infection[a]
History	Days to <3 weeks
Clinical	Pain, swelling, redness, drainage
Serology	ESR and CRP ↑
Synovial fluid WBC	+
Synovial fluid culture	+
Imaging (Plain, CT)	Stable components
Nuclear medicine	+
Management	Incision and drainage, debridement, antibiotics

Key: *ESR* Erythrocyte sedimentation rate (>30 mm/h), *CRP* C-reactive protein (>10 mg/L)
[a]Wolford et al. [35]

and ramus. A double antibiotic solution (neomycin and polymyxin B) is then irrigated through the catheters for 5 days and a peripherally inserted central catheter (PICC line) placed to deliver intravenous antibiotics based on culture and sensitivity results. On discharge from the hospital the patient is placed on the appropriate antibiotic for 4–6 weeks and monitored closely (Table 10.1). Eighty percent (4 out of 5) of patients with an acute infection in their study responded to this treatment [35].

10.4.1.2 Delayed TMJ TJR PJI

Patients presenting >3 weeks or longer after TMJ TJR with complaints increasing pain and diffuse swelling with no evidence of localized erythema, no fever and no drainage present a difficult diagnostic dilemma unless there is clinical evidence of a draining skin or auditory canal fistula directly communicating with the device. This sign is pathognomonic of a TMJ TJR PJI and requires delayed TMJ TJR infection management [30] (Table 10.2). Intrinsic causes for pain and diffuse swelling should be ruled out by imaging (plain film or CT). Since ESR and CRP can be equivocal in a late TMJ TJR infection, their value as diagnostic tests is diminished in suspected delayed TMJ TJR infection. Late infections often represent insidious biofilm infection which increases the challenge of making the correct diagnosis.

Sterile aspiration of the TMJ TJR articulation to obtain fluid for WBC analysis (>1100–4000 cells/μL; 64–68% polymorphonucleocytes) and culture is indicated. A CT scan with contrast remains the most cost-effective initial diagnostic study (Fig. 10.2).

Table 10.2 Algorithm for the management of a late TMJ TJR infection

	Late Infection[a]
History	>3 weeks to years
Clinical	Pain, swelling, ± fistula
Serology	ESR and CRP ±
Synovial fluid WBC	+
Synovial fluid culture	+
Imaging (Plain, CT)	Unstable component(s)
Nuclear medicine	+
Management	2-stage removal/replacement

Key: *ESR* Erythrocyte sedimentation rate (>30 mm/h), *CRP* C-reactive protein (>10 mg/L)
[a] Mercuri [16]

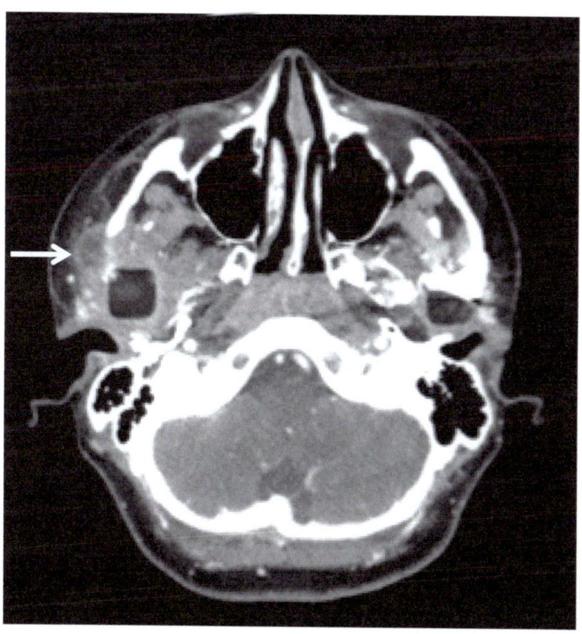

Fig. 10.2 Axial CT scan with contrast in a patient with bilateral TJR at 12 months. *White arrow* indicates small collection adjacent to the fossa component

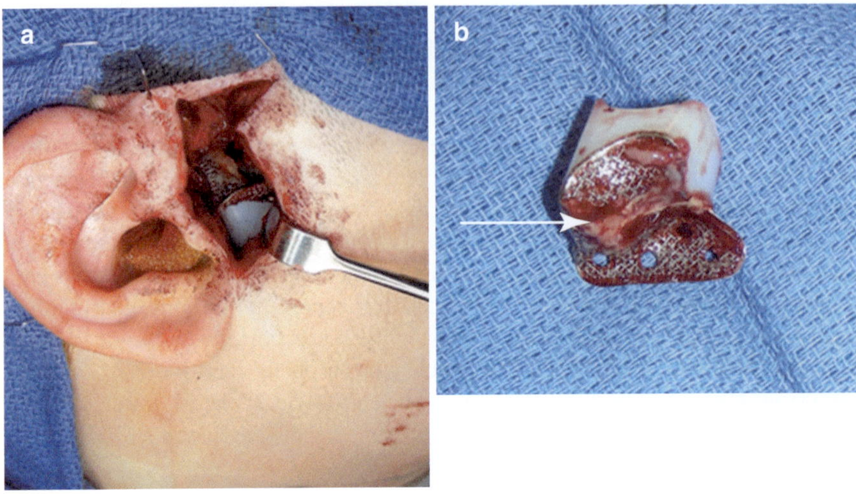

Fig. 10.3 (**a**) Removal of an MRSA infected TMJ TJR at 12 months postoperatively. (**b**) A firmly adherent biofilm on the fossa component (*white arrow*)

Labeled-leucocyte imaging (e.g., leucocytes labeled with indium-111) alone or combined with bone marrow imaging with the use of technetium-99 m–labeled sulfur colloid is considered the test of choice when nuclear imaging is utilized [37].

If a preauricular or auricular canal sinus tract is present suggesting an infection, a large endodontic gutta percha point can be inserted into the fistula and an anterior-posterior skull image made. This will demonstrate the gutta percha point in the TMJ TJR joint space indicative of a biofilm infection. Following the delayed infection management protocol (Table 10.2), the TMJ TJR device involved in the biofilm infection must be removed along with associated affected tissue. This tissue should be sent for aerobic and anaerobic culture as should any associated purulence (Fig. 10.3a, b).

Once the device components have been removed, the patient should be placed in maxillomandibular fixation, and antibiotic impregnated polymethyl methacrylate (orthopedic bone cement) should be mixed to a doughy consistence and inserted into the joint space to deliver antibiotic directly to the affected area. Appropriate antibiotic therapy, either oral or parenteral, as determined by culture and sensitivity is instituted for a period of 2–3 months [38]. It is beneficial, although not essential, to maintain the patient in maxillomandibular fixation while the antibiotic spacer is in place to avoid spacer migration or fracture and to avoid possible bony anatomical or occlusal changes with function. When it is time to replace the TMJ TJR components, the maxillomandibular fixation can be released, the antibiotic spacer removed, and the new TMJ TJR device components can be implanted [8].

Early and delayed infections are the most common cause for postimplantation pain and swelling [8, 12, 13, 15, 16]. However, if infection is ruled out, the surgeon should consider the following other common potential intrinsic and extrinsic causes for post-TMJ TJR pain. Intrinsic causes include heterotopic bone formation, dislocation, material sensitivity, aseptic component/screw loosening or fracture, osteolysis, neuroma formation, or synovial entrapment syndrome. Most of these can be diagnosed by imaging and/or diagnostic local anesthetic blocks or lab testing (i.e., lymphocyte transformation test (LTT) for metal sensitivity) and then managed appropriately with revision or replacement surgery [8].

Extrinsic causes include prior misdiagnosis, chronic centrally mediated pain, persistent myofascial/muscular pain, complex regional pain syndrome (CPRS I), neurologic injury (CPRS II), temporalis tendonitis, coronoid impingement, Frey neuralgia, and integrin formation. Extrinsic issues are the most complicated and difficult to diagnose and manage [8].

References

1. Charnley J. Low friction arthroplasty of the hip: theory and practice. Berlin: Springer-Verlag; 1979.
2. Darouiche RO. Treatment of infections associated with surgical implants. N Engl J Med. 2004;350:1422–9.
3. Zimmereli W, Trampuz A. Implant associated infection. In: Bjarnsholt T, Hoiby N, Moser C, Jensen PO, editors. Biofilm infections. 1st ed. Heidelberg: Springer; 2011. p. P69–90.
4. Salvati E, Wilson P, Jolley M. A ten-year follow-up study of our first one hundred consecutive Charnley total hip replacements. J Bone Joint Surg. 1981;63A:753–76.
5. Schulte KR, Callaghan JJ, Kelley SS, Johnston RC. The outcome of Charnley total hip arthroplasty with cement after a minimum of twenty-year follow-up. The results of one surgeon. J Bone Joint Surg. 1993;75A:961–75.
6. Sokka T, Kautiainen H, Hannonen P. Stable occurrence of knee and hip total joint replacement in Central Finland between 1986 and 2003: an indication of improved long-term outcomes of rheumatoid arthritis. Ann Rheum Dis. 2007;66:341–4.
7. Zimmereli W, Trampuz A. Biomaterial associated infection: a perspective from the clinic. In: Fintan-Moriarty T, Zaat SAJ, Busscher HJ, editors. Biomaterials associated infections. Heidelberg: Springer; 2013.
8. Mercuri LG, editor. Temporomandibular joint total joint replacement – TMJ TJR – a comprehensive reference for researchers, material scientists and surgeons. New York: Springer; 2015.
9. Kurtz SM, Ong KL, Lau E, Bozic KJ, Berry D, Parvizi J. Prosthetic joint infection risk after TKA in the Medicare population. Clin Orthop. 2010;468:52–6.
10. Ong KL, Kurtz SM, Lau E, Bozic KJ, Berry DJ, Parvizi J. Prosthetic joint infection risk after total hip arthroplasty in the Medicare population. J Arthroplasty. 2009;24(Suppl 1):105–9.
11. Kurtz SM, Ong KL, Schmier J, Mowat F, Saleh K, Dybvik E, Kärrholm J, Garellick G, Havelin LI, Furnes O, Malchau H, Lau E. Future clinical and economic impact of revision total hip and knee arthroplasty. J Bone Joint Surg Am. 2007;89(Suppl 3):144–51.
12. Mercuri LG, Psutka D. Peri-operative, post-operative and prophylactic use of antibiotics in alloplastic total temporomandibular joint replacement surgery: a survey and preliminary guidelines. J Oral Maxillofac Surg. 2011;69:2106–11.
13. Mercuri LG. Temporomandibular joint replacement periprosthetic joint infections: a review of early diagnostic testing options. Int J Oral Maxillofac Surg. 2014;43:1236–42.
14. Lima ALL, Oliveira PR, Carvalho VC, Saconi ES, Cabrita HB, Rodrigues MB. Periprosthetic joint infections. Interdiscip Perspect Infect Dis. 2013;2013:542796. doi:10.1155/2013/542796.. Epub 2013 Aug 19.

15. Mercuri LG. Microbial biofilms – a potential source of alloplastic device failure. J Oral Maxillofac Surg. 2006;64:1303–9.
16. Mercuri LG. Avoiding and managing temporomandibular joint total joint replacement surgical site infections. J Oral Maxillofac Surg. 2012;70:2280–9.
17. Gordon A, Greenfield EM, Eastell R, Kiss-Toth E, Wilkinson JM. Individual susceptibility to periprosthetic osteolysis is associated with altered patterns of innate immune gene expression in response to pro-inflammatory stimuli. J Orthop Res. 2010;28:1127–35.
18. Cooper RA. Surgical site infections: epidemiology and microbiological aspects in trauma and orthopedic surgery. Int Wound J. 2013;10(Suppl 1):3–8.
19. Kagansky N, Berner Y, Koren-Morag N, Perelman L, Knobler H, Levy S. Poor nutritional habits are predictors of poor outcome in very old hospitalized patients. Am J Clin Nutr. 2005;2:784–91.
20. Sørensen LT. Wound healing and infection in surgery. The clinical impact of smoking and smoking cessation: a systematic review and meta-analysis. Arch Surg. 2012;147:373–83.
21. Møller AM, Villebro N, Pedersen T, Tønnesen H. Effect of preoperative smoking intervention on postoperative complications: a randomized clinical trial. Lancet. 2002;359:114–7.
22. Wong J, Lam DP, Abrishami A, Chan MT, Chung F. Short-term preoperative smoking cessation and postoperative complications: a systematic review and meta-analysis. Can J Anaesth. 2012;59:268–79.
23. Sørensen LT, Karlsmark T, Gottrup F. Abstinence from smoking reduces incisional wound infection: a randomized controlled trial. Ann Surg. 2003;238:1–5.
24. Edwards LD. The epidemiology of 2056 remote site infections and 1966 surgical wound infections occurring in 1865 patients: a four-year study of 40, 923 operations at Rush-Presbyterian-St. Luke's Hospital, Chicago. Ann Surg. 1976;184:758–66.
25. Uçkay I, Pittet D, Bernard L, Lew D, Perrier A, Peter R. Antibiotic prophylaxis before invasive dental procedures in patients with arthroplasties of the hip and knee. J Bone Joint Surg Br. 2008;90:833–8.
26. Webster J, Osborne S. Preoperative bathing or showering with skin antiseptics to prevent surgical site infection. Cochrane Database Syst Rev. 2007;(18):CD004985.
27. Mangram AJ, Horan TC, Pearson ML, Silver LC, Jarvis WR. Guideline for prevention of surgical site infection, 1999. Centers for Disease Control and Prevention (CDC) Hospital Infection Control Practices Advisory Committee. Am J Infect Control. 1999;27:97–132.
28. Rosenberg AD, Wambold D, Kraemer L, Begley-Keyes M, Zuckerman SL, Singh N, Cohen MM, Bennett MV. Ensuring appropriate timing of antimicrobial prophylaxis. J Bone Joint Surg Am. 2008;90:226–32.
29. Levent T, Vandevelde D, Delobelle JM, Labourdette P, Létendard J, Lesage P, Lecocq P, Dufour M. Infection risk prevention following total knee arthroplasty. Orthop Traumatol Surg Res. 2010;96:48–56.
30. Mercuri LG. Total reconstruction of the temporomandibular joint with a custom system. In: Ness G, editor. Atlas of oral and maxillofacial clinics of North America. Current concepts in temporomandibular joint surgery. Philadelphia: Elsevier Saunders; 2011. p. 233–42.
31. Towfigh S, Cheadle WG, Lowry SF, Malangoni MA, Wilson SE. Significant reduction in incidence of wound contamination by skin flora through use of microbial sealant. Arch Surg. 2008;143:885–91.
32. Cheung EV, Sperling JW, Cofield RH. Infection associated with hematoma formation after shoulder arthroplasty. Clin Orthop Relat Res. 2008;466:1363–7.
33. Zmistowski B, Restrepo C, Kahl LK, Parvizi J, Sharkey PF. Incidence and reasons for nonrevision reoperation after total knee arthroplasty. Clin Orthop Relat Res. 2011;469:138–45.
34. de Beer J, Petruccelli D, Rotstein C, Weening B, Royston K, Winemaker M. Antibiotic prophylaxis for total joint replacement surgery: results of a survey of Canadian orthopedic surgeons. Can J Surg. 2009;52:E229–34.
35. Wolford LM, Rodrigues DB, McPhillips A. Management of the infected temporomandibular joint total joint prosthesis. J Oral Maxillofac Surg. 2010;68:2810–23.

36. Della Valle C, Parvizi J, Bauer TW, DiCesare PE, Evans RP, Segreti J, Spangehi M. The diagnosis of periprosthetic joint infections of the hip and knee. Guideline and evidence report. Adopted by the American Academy of Orthopedic Surgeons. Rosemont: American Academy of Orthopedic Surgeons; 2010.
37. Love C, Marwin SE, Palestro CJ. Nuclear medicine and the infected joint replacement. Semin Nucl Med. 2009;39:66–70.
38. Berend KR, Lombardi Jr AV, Morris MJ, Bergeson AG, Adams JB, Sneller MA. Two-stage treatment of hip periprosthetic joint infection is associated with a high rate of infection control but high mortality. Clin Orthop Relat Res. 2013;471:510–8.

Iatrogenic Degenerative Joint Disease

11

Joseph P. McCain and Alexandra G. Glickman

The most important consideration in the treatment of the temporomandibular joint dysfunction (TMD) patient is making a proper diagnosis and selecting an appropriate treatment using evidence-based guidelines and algorithms. The approach to treatment should include strategies to educate the patient about their disease process, the current stage of that disease, how to manage it, and preventative approaches to reduce the likelihood of disease progression. Diet and lifestyle changes play an important role in the management of TMD just as they do in many other systemic diseases. When combined with appropriate surgical intervention in the properly selected patient, outcomes can be better predicted with the potential to slow or prevent the development of internal derangement.

Irrespective of the stage of internal derangement or the presence of degenerative joint disease, conservative treatment generally results in more than 90% of patients substantially improving. In those who fail to respond to conservative treatment and who are deemed appropriate candidates for surgical intervention, the success rates approach 80–90%. Success has most commonly been defined as a reduction in pain, improved maximum incisal opening (MIO), and improved jaw function using one of several validated scales. It is important to continually assess patient responses to both conservative and surgical treatment. Simple questionnaires to record pain, MIO, and function are easy and convenient to administer at each patient appointment (Fig. 11.1).

J.P. McCain, DMD, FACS (✉)
Voluntary Clinical Professor and Chief Oral & Maxillofacial Surgery,
Florida International University, Herbert Wertheim School of Medicine, Miami, FL, USA
e-mail: jmccain@miamioms.com

A.G. Glickman, DDS
Hudson Valley Oral Surgery, New York, Fishkill, NY, USA

Endoscopic Oral and Maxillofacial Surgery, Miami, FL, USA

G.F. Bouloux (ed.), *Complications of Temporomandibular Joint Surgery*,
DOI 10.1007/978-3-319-51241-9_11

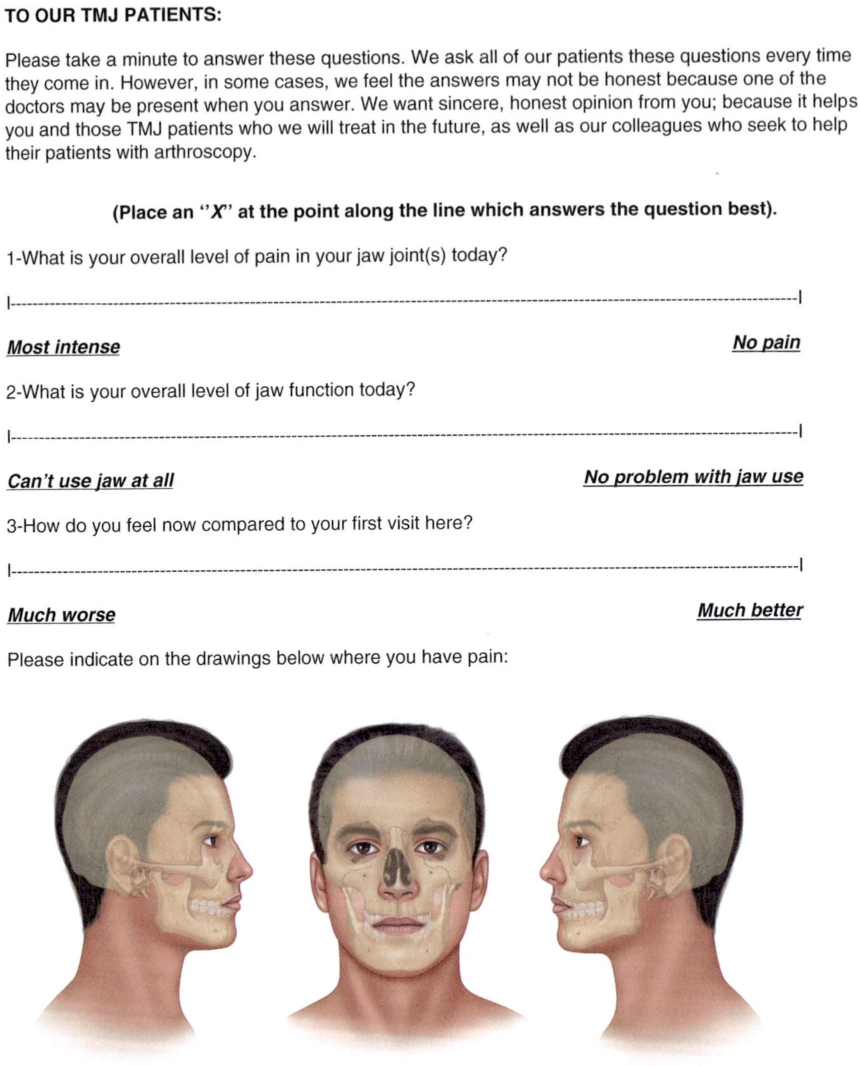

Fig. 11.1 Patient reported data

The primary goal of surgical intervention is to reduce joint inflammation and pain, improve joint function, and reduce the likelihood of disease progression. Despite an appropriate surgical intervention, disease progression may occur in some patients necessitating further treatment, including additional surgery. This does not mean that the original surgical procedure was a failure as delaying any additional surgery while improving pain and function is a reasonable goal. The potential for degenerative joint disease (DJD) to develop or progress over time following arthroscopy or arthroplasty remains a challenge. Despite this fact, postsurgical remodeling following surgical intervention is expected and may often result in satisfactory clinical outcomes irrespective of radiographic DJD.

Table 11.1 Etiology of TMJ pathology

Etiology	Example
Parafunction	Direct microtrauma (associated MPD, bruxism and clenching)
Dentofacial deformity and malocclusion	Direct microtrauma (most commonly in vertical maxillary excess patients with mandibular retrognathia, Class II patients)
Direct macrotrauma	Direct trauma to the mandible with or without fracture, sometimes evidenced by well-defined scar on patient chin
Indirect macrotrauma	Acceleration-deceleration type phenomenon
Systemic disease	Immunologic diseases, benign or malignant tumors

Iatrogenic causes of temporomandibular joint disease and pathology may be the result of several factors. The most basic is the failure to make the correct diagnosis. The second relates to the choice of an inappropriate procedure given the diagnosis and patient-specific psychological and social factors. The third relates to the failure to establish realistic patient and surgeon expectations. The last relates to procedural specific issues including the use of intra-articular medications, instrumentation during surgical procedures, bleeding, and vascular compromise. The latter may result in chondromalacia, DJD, bleeding, adhesion formation, ankylosis, and condylar resorption with the potential for decreased function and persistent pain.

It is imperative that all patients are approached in a systematic way that allows the surgeon to make the correct diagnosis, identify contributing factors, and develop a treatment strategy that is patient centered. The initial visit should consist of a thorough clinical examination, a history that asks a series of very pointed questions, and evaluating plain film (panoramic) imaging to make the correct diagnosis. There are generally five broad causes of TMD that should be considered. Responses to treatment will ultimately depend on many factors including the etiology of the patient's disease process (Table 11.1).

Tradition dictates that the chief complaint and history of the present illness be obtained initially. This ultimately allows a focused physical examination. Contrary to this dogma, the authors have found that performing a physical examination prior to engaging in a conversation with the patient is more beneficial as it obviates any bias related to subjective complaints. This should not be misconstrued to suggest that the findings of an isolated physical examination are more likely to result in the correct diagnosis as ultimately this also requires a thorough history and imaging. The key components to the physical examination include the patient at rest, opening and closing position, velocity of opening, end opening, lateral and protrusive excursions, MIO, and joint loading (Fig. 11.2a–f). An evaluation of the panoramic film follows which allows for degenerative joint disease, condylar resorption, and other osseous pathology to be recognized (Fig. 11.3). A focused history can then be obtained to include the location and duration of the pain, functional limitations, and activities that either increase or decrease the pain.

At the initial consultation, surgery is rarely discussed unless there is a clear indication (e.g., closed lock with failed conservative management, bony ankylosis).

Initial advice consists of the standard conservative treatment including avoiding daytime clenching, diet modification, and nocturnal splint use. Nonsteroidal anti-inflammatory medications and muscle relaxants for a period of time may also be indicated depending on the diagnosis and stage of the disease. If a patient is suspected of having concomitant myofascial or cervical pain, then referral to a physical therapist is required.

For the experienced temporomandibular joint surgeon, the correct diagnosis, etiology, and future treatment can mostly be formulated during the initial consultation. In a majority of patients, a short course of conservative therapy in those patients who have not been through this modality yet is recommended. Conservative treatment while controlling parafunctional habits (if present) will result in a substantial

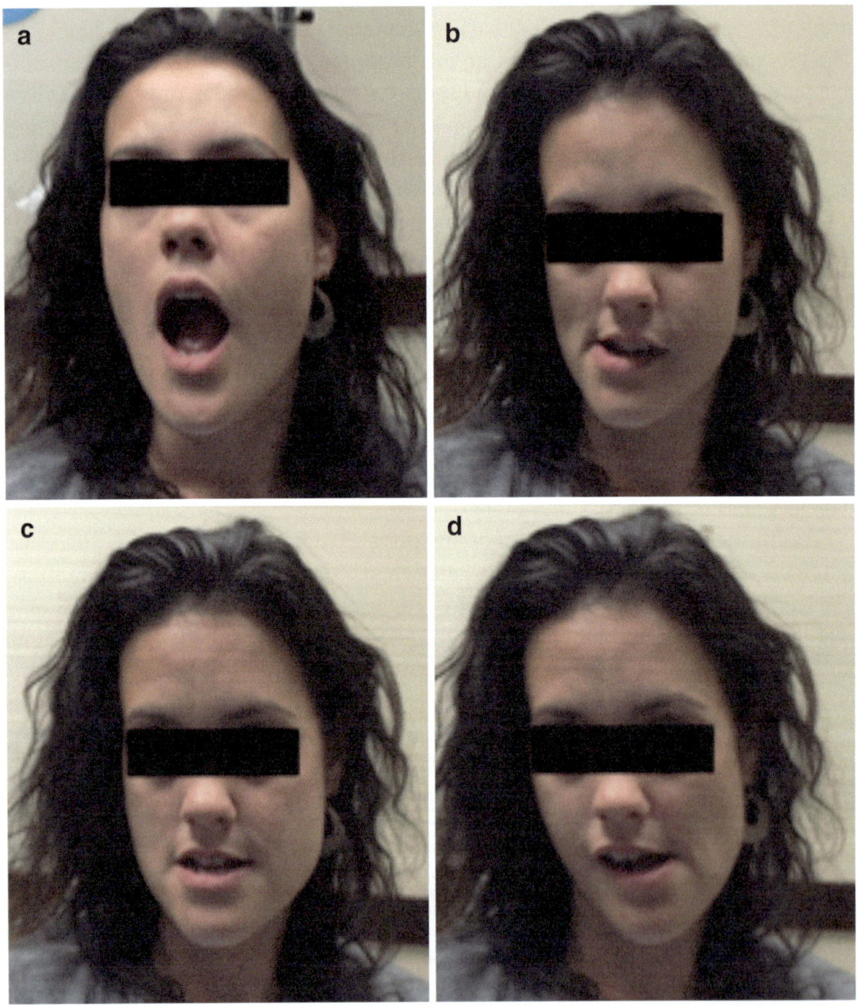

Fig. 11.2 (**a**) Maximum incisal opening. (**b**) Right lateral excursion. (**c**) Protrusion. (**d**) Left lateral excursion. (**e**) Mahan test (left side). (**f**) Mahan test (right side)

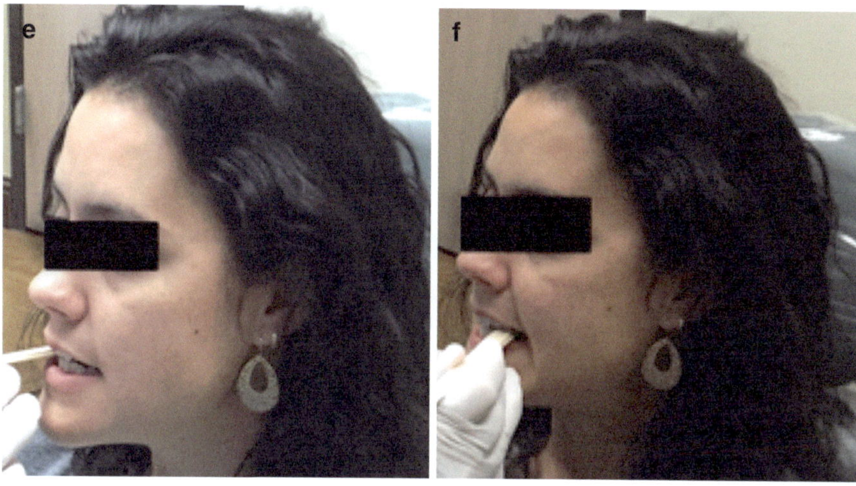

Fig. 11.2 (continued)

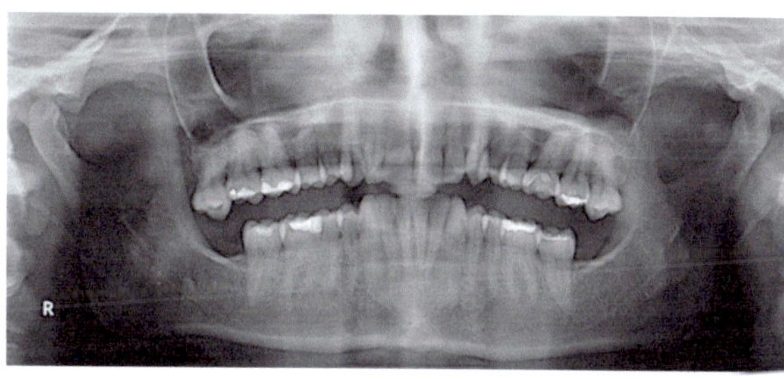

Fig. 11.3 Panoramic imaging

improvement in the majority of patients. Additionally it will provide the opportunity for the surgeon to get to know the patient and learn of any psychological, social, or comorbid conditions that may affect the response to treatment, including surgery.

Patients that are deemed to be surgical candidates subsequently require additional diagnostic testing to determine more specifically the diagnosis and an appropriate treatment plan. Generally speaking temporomandibular joint disorders can be divided into the two broad categories of inflammatory arthritis and noninflammatory arthrosis. This helps provide a basic algorithm to guide subsequent surgical intervention (Fig. 11.4).

Inflammatory disorders may be divided into primary or secondary arthritis. The common denominator in all inflammatory arthritis would appear to be synovitis. Primary arthritides include local and systemic diseases with a strong specific immunologic mechanism. Any single joint can be involved including the TMJ although it is more common to involve multiple joints. Additional bodily systems may also be involved depending on the disease. Establishing the correct diagnosis in these patients can be a challenge. It is recommended that prior to any surgical decision-making, serology be performed (Table 11.2). This should include rheumatoid factor, cyclic citrullinated peptide antibody, antinuclear antibody, and human leukocyte antigen B27. It is also recommended to evaluate the vitamin D and 17B-estradiol

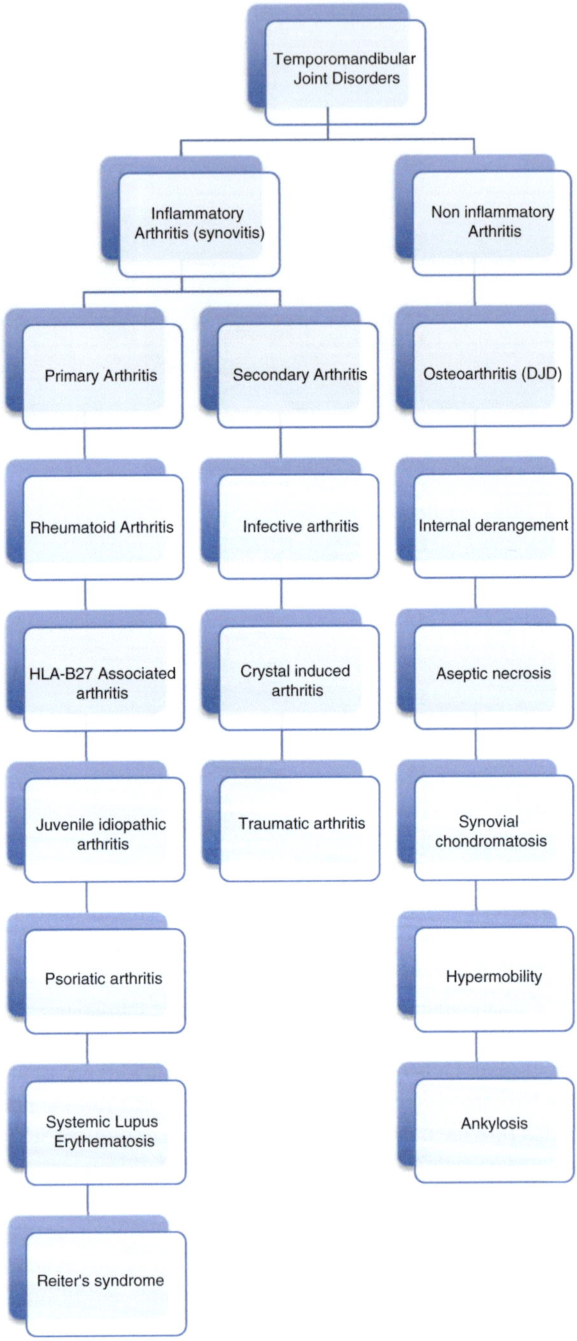

Fig. 11.4 Classification system for intra-articular pathology

Table 11.2 Serology and laboratory tests

Lab test	Disease
Rheumatoid factor	Rheumatoid arthritis
Cyclic citrullinated peptide antibody	Rheumatoid arthritis
Antinuclear antibody	Rheumatoid arthritis, systemic lupus erythematosis
HLA B27	Reiter's syndrome, reactive arthritis, ankylosing spondylitis
Vitamin D	Bone remodeling
17B-estradiol	Progressive condylar resorption

levels as 17B-estradiol receptors have been isolated in the TMJ and, in excess, have been associated with condylar resorption. Identifying the likely etiology of the inflammatory response within the TMJ remains vital to the overall success of their treatment. If one neglects to identify a rheumatologic disorder, any proposed surgical intervention while possibly resulting in a positive short-term outcome will likely result in treatment failure in the long term. If the results of serology suggest an inflammatory arthritide, the patient should be referred to the rheumatologist for further evaluation and medical management. If the patient's symptoms persist despite optimized rheumatologic medical management, then they may enter the surgical treatment algorithm in the same manner a patient without rheumatologic disease would.

Secondary arthritides include reactive infective arthritis, traumatic arthritis, and crystal-induced arthritis (gout, pseudogout). Reactive infective arthritis has been identified as a result of chlamydia trachomatis (42%), mycoplasma fermentans/orale (23%), and mycoplasma genitalium (35%) [1]. The clinical importance remains controversial although there may be a benefit to submitting a small synovial biopsy specimen for polymerase chain reaction (PCR) to determine if bacterial DNA is present. Crystal-induced arthropathy is extremely rare in the temporomandibular joint. The diagnosis is typically only made during arthroscopy or open surgery when the joint is explored and "crystals" are found. There appears to be little benefit in measuring serum calcium and uric acid given the extremely low incidence of crystal arthropathy within the temporomandibular joint.

Noninflammatory arthritis is generally considered to have less inflammation than the inflammatory arthritides and result from excessive mechanical loading with the production of reactive oxygen species and oxidative stress ultimately leading to DJD [2]. The presence of inflammatory mediators and degraded proteins has been well documented within temporomandibular joint lavage fluid [3–9]. Additionally, the concentration of these mediators and the degree to which they are removed following arthrocentesis and arthroscopy correlates with both initial symptoms and the response to treatment, respectively [10]. Although joint inflammation appears to play a role in the development and persistence of joint pain and reduced function in most patients, there is a subset of patients in whom disc position appears to be critical. Internal derangement is most often classified using Wilkes criteria (Table 11.3). Discopexy and discectomy with or without replacement may be appropriate procedures in these patients.

Table 11.3 Wilkes classification

Stage	Findings
I	Anterior disc displacement with reduction. No pain and locking
II	Anterior disc displacement with reduction. Pain and occasional locking
III	Anterior disc displacement without reduction. Pain and closed lock may be present
IV	Anterior disc displacement without reduction with degenerative joint disease. Pain is present
V	Anterior disc displacement without reduction with degenerative joint disease. Pain and crepitation is present

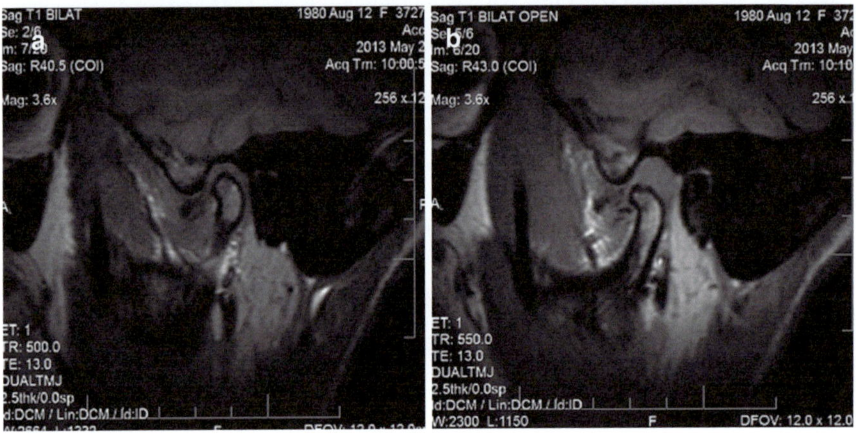

Fig. 11.5 (**a**) T1-weighted right TMJ closed sagittal MRI. (**b**) T1-weighted right TMJ open sagittal MRI

If considering a surgical procedure, advanced imaging becomes increasingly important. Magnetic resonance imaging (MRI) of the bilateral temporomandibular joints to identify disc position, disc morphology, medullary and cortical bone, presence of an effusion, and joint dynamics remains the standard. The MRI should be without contrast on a 1.5 Tesla coiled machine (Fig. 11.5a, b). Further bone-specific imaging with a computed tomography (CT) or a cone-beam computed tomogram (CBCT) may also be beneficial to evaluate joint space and bone morphology (Fig. 11.6).

After completion of the examination, history taking, and imaging, the patient should be ready to enter an appropriate surgical algorithm. However, it can be difficult to identify the correct diagnosis in some patients even after all of the above testing has been completed. In these situations, the authors advocate diagnostic arthroscopy. The importance of obtaining the correct diagnosis and controlling etiological factors cannot be underestimated when contemplating surgical procedures in order to obtain and maintain a positive outcome.

A surgical armamentarium for the treatment of the temporomandibular joint includes arthrocentesis, arthroscopy (levels I, II, III), arthroplasty with disc plication

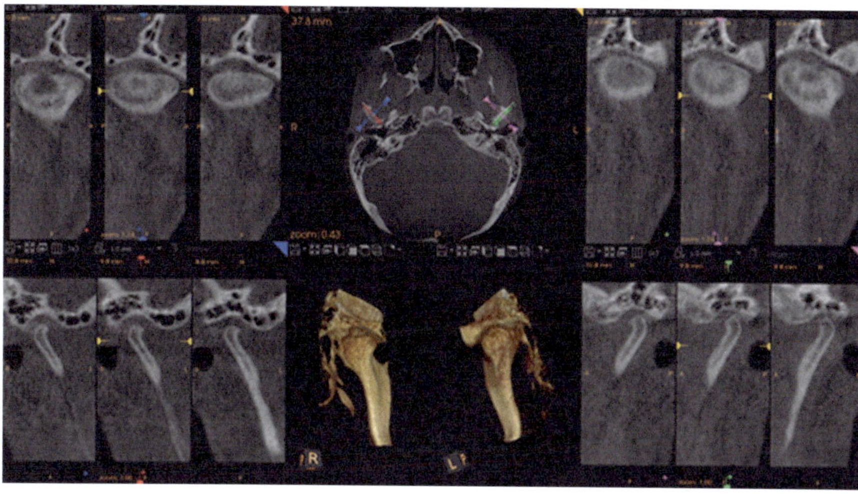

Fig. 11.6 Cone beam computed tomography (CBCT)

or discectomy, and total joint replacement. The need for disc replacement following discectomy remains controversial although the authors favor replacement.

11.1 Arthrocentesis and Arthroscopy

Arthrocentesis or arthroscopy should be considered for the majority of patients with TMJ pain or dysfunction. Bony ankylosis, advanced fibrous ankylosis, and ankylosing osteoarthritis preclude this approach and require arthroplasty. The authors prefer arthroscopy over arthrocentesis as it is both diagnostic and therapeutic for patients who have pain and dysfunction providing the opportunity for visualization of joint structures as well as biopsy and instrumentation.

11.1.1 Arthrocentesis

Indications for arthrocentesis include patients with anchored disc phenomenon and Wilkes grade II, III, and early IV. It can be performed under local anesthesia, intravenous sedation in the office, or in the operating room under general anesthesia. Its goal is to decrease pain and increase range of motion through lavage of the joint with removal of inflammatory mediators and degraded proteins. It can also potentially disrupt an anchored disc and allow the instillation of medication [11].

The technique is simple with the patient seated at a 45 degree angle. The location of the needle puncture sites is based on the tragal-canthal line, with the posterior puncture site 10 mm anterior to the tragus and 2 mm below the line and the anterior puncture site 20 mm anterior and 10 mm below the line. Variations on this technique exist. Prior to placing the posterior needle, the joint is insufflated with 2–3 mL of local anesthetic, and then the lavage needles are placed in position to maintain a patent fluid path. The ideal volume and medium for lavage is usually 60–350 cc of lactated ringer's solution with the amount of irrigation varying from author to author. Generally, 50 cc of LR is adequate to remove more than 95% of inflammatory mediators, while 200 cc suffices to remove more than 95% of degraded collagen, elastin, proteoglycans, and HA [10]. After lavage, the anterior needle port is removed, and the posterior port may be used to inject medication if desired. Subsequently, the patient is manipulated under anesthesia to duplicate normal joint rotation and translation. There is an overall success rate of approximately 70% for patients in whom this procedure was performed.

Although the simplicity of the procedure is appealing, arthrocentesis does not enhance diagnosis or facilitate biopsy. Additionally the procedure cannot disrupt restrictive adhesions, particularly when mature. Furthermore, there is little opportunity to educate the patient about the diagnosis or prognosis. Complications are exceedingly rare with arthrocentesis; however, great care is required during the procedure to avoid scuffing the fossa and creating an area of chondromalacia that was not previously present.

Variations in this procedure revolve around the types of medications that can be injected into the joint at the completion of the procedure. Hyaluronic acid (HA), steroids, and, most recently, platelet-rich plasma (PRP) have all been advocated. The science guiding the choice of medication is generally weak. Selecting an appropriate medication should be based on the patient profile and preoperative diagnosis. When these medications are injected during arthrocentesis, they are released into the entirety of the superior joint compartment. In the event that the joint is a Wilkes V, they are released into both the superior joint space and the inferior joint space as they are connected by the disc perforation. As a result all joint structures are subject to action by the medication including the condyle in cases of disc perforation.

Hyaluronic acid has been shown to reduce inflammation, enhance lubrication, and promote cartilage repair without any deleterious effects on joint tissues following arthroscopy [12]. The use of HA in severely inflamed joints is contraindicated as a result of the potential for an acute flare of symptoms. As arthrocentesis is a blind procedure and does not permit the recognition of inflammation within the joint, the use of HA following arthrocentesis may not be appropriate.

The use of steroid injections has proven to be somewhat controversial. Typical steroids that can be injected into the joint include dexamethasone, triamcinolone acetonide, and betamethasone. Long-acting triamcinolone hexacetonide is no longer available in the USA despite its popularity in rheumatology. All steroids result in a reduction of inflammation and hence pain. The short-term effect in reducing joint inflammation and pain has been reported, particularly in the pediatric population diagnosed with juvenile idiopathic arthritis. Despite an initial reduction in inflammation, there is concern that repeated injections will incite condylar resorption or retard growth in this important center of the facial skeleton. The potential to hasten joint degradation in both cartilage and bone has been documented in other joints [13]. Steroids should not be the first choice for use in noninflammatory arthropathy but may play a role in the management of patients with primary inflammatory arthropathy. Current evidence suggests that neither HA nor steroids are superior to arthrocentesis alone in noninflammatory conditions within the TMJ [14, 15].

Platelet-rich plasma (PRP) has been used in oral and maxillofacial surgery for mandibular reconstruction. Platelet-rich plasma concentrates the seven fundamental growth factors secreted by platelets to begin the wound healing process, and in so doing it promotes healing. The use in orthopedic surgery corroborated this hypothesis by showing the reversal of deleterious effects of osteoarthritis on articular cartilage [16]. A meta-analysis of arthroscopic knee surgery showed a significant improvement in pain and function when compared to HA [17]. A beneficial effect of PRP has also been demonstrated following arthrocentesis although long-term data is lacking [18]. The role of PRP in treating TMJ pain and osteoarthritis remains unclear until further studies are completed.

At the present time, the most ideal medications to use in arthrocentesis are not clear. It seems reasonable to avoid any adjunct medications in patients with noninflammatory DJD and use steroids judiciously in patients with inflammatory arthropathy. The use of PRP, while promising, has little evidence to support or refute its use.

11.1.2 Arthroscopy

Arthroscopic surgery has evolved significantly since it was first introduced by Ohnishi. It is a very safe and minimally invasive way to provide many levels of treatment on patients who would historically require open surgical techniques with much higher complication rates. The most important indication for diagnostic and operative arthroscopy is pain and dysfunction that cannot be reversed through conservative measures. Regardless of disease stage, it allows the surgeon to make a diagnosis through direct visualization of the joint, simultaneously perform lavage, manipulate structures (e.g., break adhesions), take biopsies, and thoroughly debride or reconstruct the joint as indicated by the preoperative and intraoperative diagnosis. Absolute contraindications to arthroscopy include bony ankylosis, preauricular skin infection, or preauricular tumor.

Arthroscopy is performed at three different surgical levels based on the diagnosis and surgeon experience. Level I is a single posterolateral puncture technique where the scope is introduced and a diagnostic sweep completed to visualize all important structures and a patent irrigation portal is maintained to lavage the joint. Level II is a double-puncture technique with an additional anterolateral puncture site for passageway of instrumentation. Level IIIa is a double or triple puncture technique, which allows for scope entry in the posterior port and large diameter instrumentation in an anterior port for advanced debridement or partial meniscectomy in end-stage disease. Level IIIb is a reconstructive arthroscopy whereby an arthroscopic discopexy is completed.

In performing this procedure, patient preparation and correct positioning are paramount. The patient's preauricular surgical site should be parallel to the floor so that the operator has the advantage of recognizing all anatomical landmarks. An ear wick should be in place to avoid otologic injury. Each step is carefully designed to maintain the safety of the procedure and to obtain more information about the joint space. First, the intra and extra-articular landmarks must be identified via manipulation of the jaw. Then while the mandible is distracted, 2% lidocaine in a 3.5 cc syringe with a 27 g needle is injected into the joint for insufflation from an inferolateral approach until 0.5 cc rebound is achieved (Fig. 11.7a).

After insufflation, the first puncture is placed at the maximum concavity of the glenoid fossa (Fig. 11.7b). Every puncture into the joint is incredibly technique sensitive as this is when the surgeon can cause significant iatrogenic damage to the joint if not executed properly. The trocar is rotated carefully through subcutaneous tissues until it reaches the lateral aspect of temporal bone; then it is used as a periosteal elevator to release the periosteum before gently sliding into the glenoid fossa and superior joint space. The maximum entry length of the trocar should never pass 25 mm measured from the surface of the integument or this can violate the structures medial to the joint capsule such as the middle ear. The authors cannot stress how important this puncture is in the success of this procedure. If not performed properly, it can lead to damage to adjacent structures and iatrogenic injury to the fibrocartilage and bone of the joint, and additionally, with multiple punctures this can lead to extravasation of fluid making it incredibly difficult to maintain any insufflation for the rest of the procedure.

Once inside the joint, the trocar is removed and the joint is gently backwashed with lactated ringer's solution and 1:300,000 epinephrine to remove any clot before inserting the scope. This irrigating fluid is used for the remainder of the case. To establish a patent outflow system, the surgeon inserts a 22 gauge 1.5 inch needle approximately 5 mm anterior and 5 mm inferior from the scope port. Then the procedure can commence with an initial lavage which is completed with 120 cc of irrigating fluid (Fig. 11.7c). Once completed, the operator should perform the diagnostic sweep to evaluate all seven points of interest in the superior joint space for abnormal pathology including disc position, degeneration of structures, or inflammatory markers (Fig. 11.7d). After reaching the anterior recess, the operator can inject medication and conclude the procedure. The authors prefer to inject hyaluronic acid for Wilkes II–IV and PRP for Wilkes V stage patients.

If the operator is to continue to level II arthroscopy, a second port needs to be obtained. This is placed in the most anterior lateral aspect of the joint to ensure maximum flexibility of the instrumentation passed through it. The puncture site is identified using triangulation principles with the scope in the anterior recess focused on the most anterior lateral aspect of the joint space. The vectors of instrument orientation here create an equilateral triangle, facilitating a repeatable and safe pattern of placement for second puncture. The depth of the arthroscope is assessed from the cannula. While the scope is held still, attention is drawn back

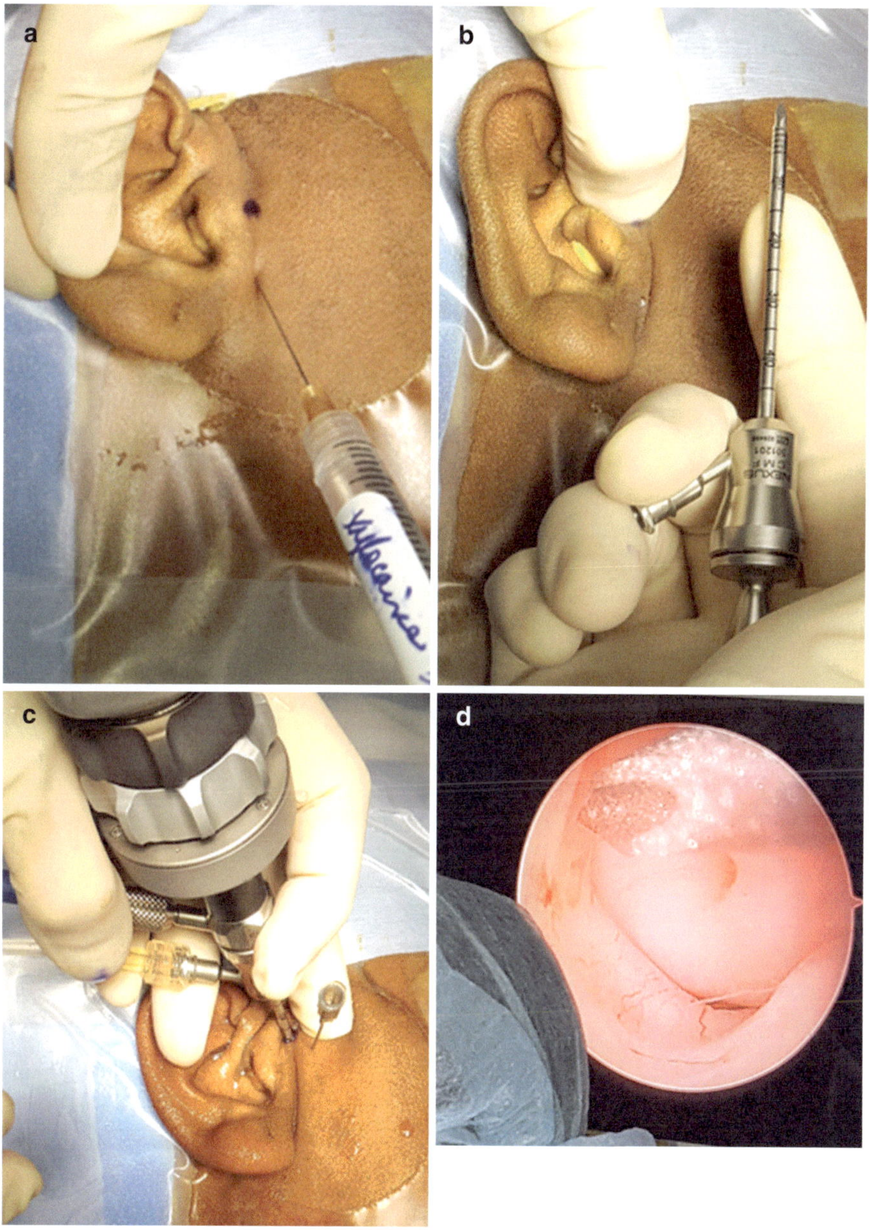

Fig. 11.7 (a) Insufflation with local anesthetic. (b) Trocar and sharp cannula. (c) Level I arthroscopy with arthroscope and irrigating needle. (d) Triangulating and identification of irrigating needle

to the skin, and a measuring cannula is laid flat against the skin with the tip (0 mm marking) in contact with the scope at point of entry while the depth of penetration is translated to this measuring cannula for a second port site (Fig. 11.8a). While the assistant insufflates the joint, the operator uses first an irrigating needle to sound the position of the port and subsequently removes it to place the trocar in the same confirmed position. This limits the amount of injury to structures inside the joint and creates less extravasation, as the needle is 22 gauge diameter compared to the 2.0 mm diameter of the cannula. The trocar is then rotated through skin and advanced at the same angulation as the irrigating needle was placed under direct visualization of the scope so that again no intra-articular structures are injured (Fig. 11.8b).

At this stage of the operation, several Level II procedures can be performed including synovial biopsy, disc manipulation, minor debridement, and contracture (Fig. 11.9a, b). In level II procedures, a contracture can be performed to tighten the lax retrodiscal tissues of a dislocated disc. Contracture can be performed via chemical (sclerosing agent) or mechanical means. The authors do not advocate the use of chemical contracture because even though it is targeted in the retrodiscal tissue, the potential for compromising the vascular supply and initiating condylar resorption or DJD exists. Contracture by mechanical means, however, is a safe and successful procedure in Wilkes II, III, and IV patients. It is performed using coblation or laser. The coblation or laser must target the redundant retrodiscal tissues, oblique protuberance, and superficial vasculature to obtain maximum effect. It is imperative that the surgeon understand and identify the appropriate intra-articular landmarks prior to contracture.

Level IIIa debridement can be achieved simply by switching out the 2.0 s puncture cannula for a 3.0 system to clean joints with arthrofibrosis, synovial

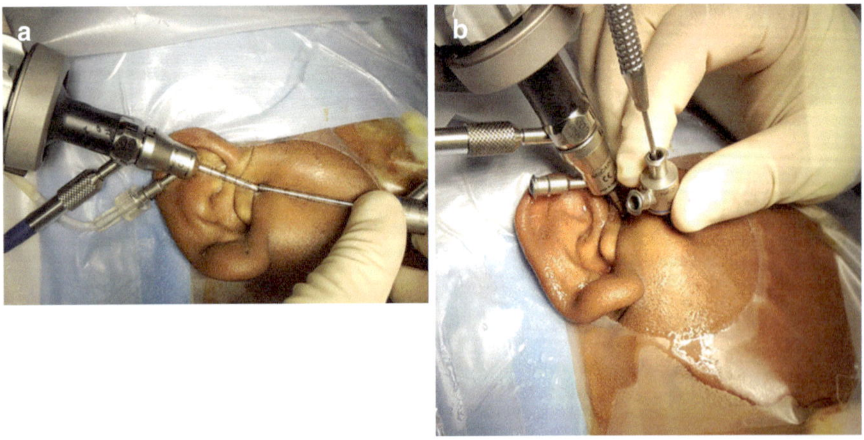

Fig. 11.8 (**a**) Level II arthroscopy with triangulation to identify second puncture site. (**b**) Level II arthroscopy with instrumentation

hyperplasia, chondromalacia stages III and IV, and ankylosing osteoarthritis (Fig. 11.10a–d). It is best to start in the anterior recess and work to the posterior by opening and increasing joint space. Debridement is achieved using hand instrumentation such as curettes or bone files, holmium laser, motorized mini shavers and abraders, coblation therapy, bipolar and monopolar electrocautery, and suction punches. Level III procedures should only be performed by experienced arthroscopic surgeons.

Historically, the most common complication of arthroscopy is iatrogenic scuffing of the fibrocartilage covering the eminence and fossa because every step beginning with insufflation is aimed to reach the maximum concavity of the glenoid fossa

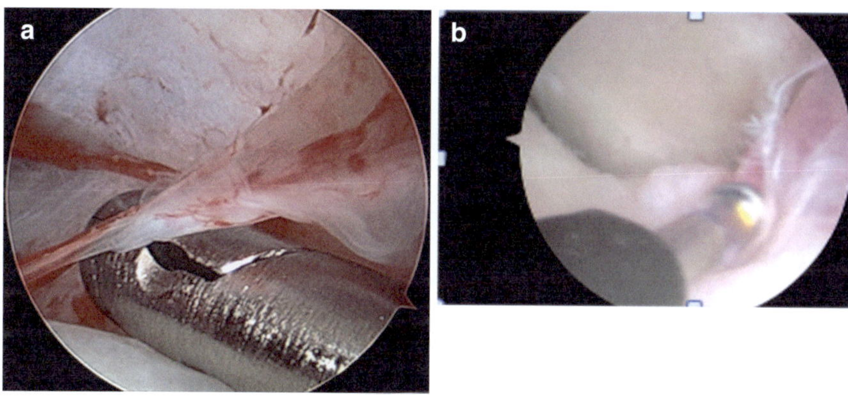

Fig. 11.9 (**a**) Arthroscopic synovial biopsy. (**b**) Arthroscopic coblation to create mechanical contracture

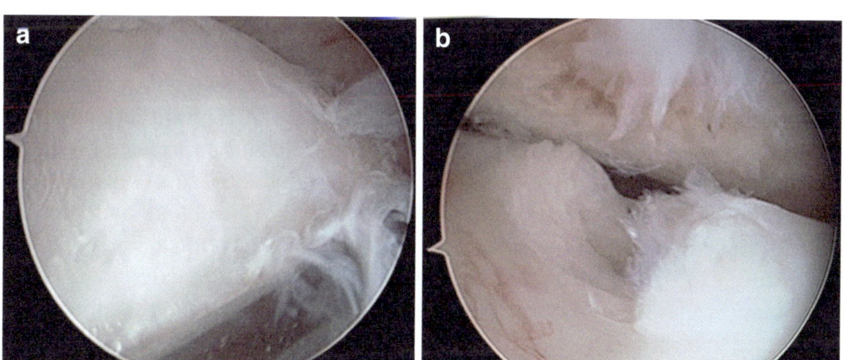

Fig. 11.10 (**a**) Grade III chondromalacia. (**b**) Grade IV chondromalacia. (**c**) Fibrous adhesion, chondromalacia, synovitis, and plicae. (**d**) Grade IV chondromalacia and perforation. (*A* backslope of the eminence, *B* chondromalacia, *C* condylar head, *D* edge of disc perforation)

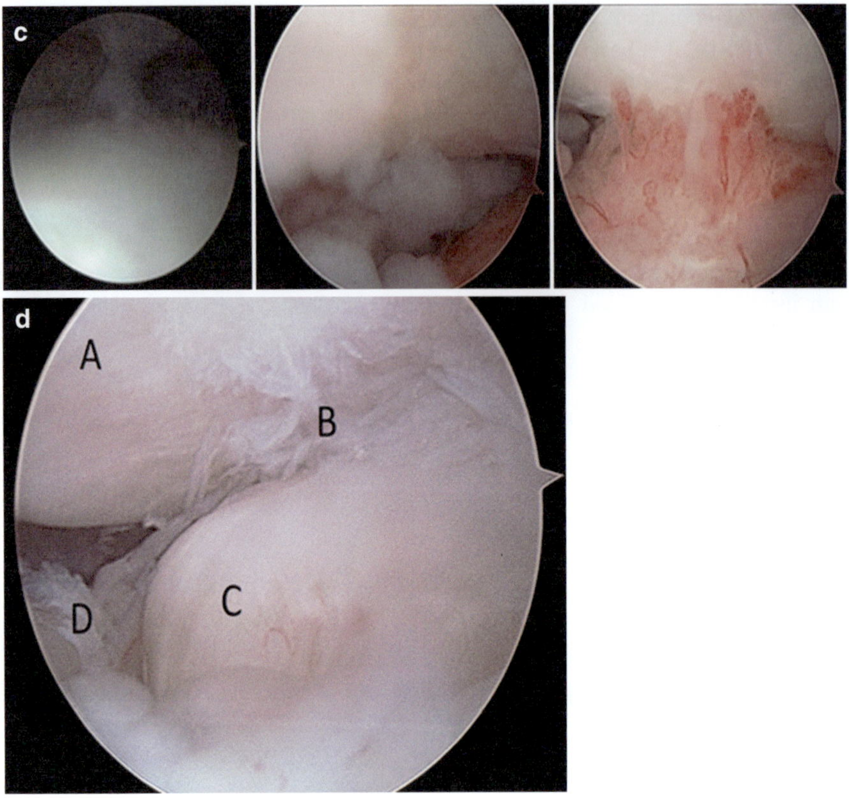

Fig. 11.10 (continued)

(Fig. 11.11a, b). During insufflation, the tip of the needle is directed toward the posterior slope of the eminence, making contact with the fibrocartilage to confirm anatomic position prior to deposition. If performed more than once, and with hasty hand, it can result in scuffing of the articulating surfaces of the fossa. After insufflation, the first puncture involves elevating the periosteum over the lateral aspect of the zygomatic arch and penetrating the capsule at the greatest concavity of the fossa with the sharp trocar. If this is not positioned correctly and is too anterior, it can scuff and injure the posterior slope of the eminence and if it is done with too much force, it can scuff the fibrocartilage of the glenoid fossa or even puncture into the middle cranial fossa. Arthroscopic cadaver studies have shown the incidence of minor scuffing of the articular surface to be between 36 and 50% [19–21]. It follows that the goal is to avoid or minimize scuffing in order to maximize the success of the procedure. Although fibrocartilage has some limited self-reparative properties through regeneration of collagen and proteoglycans, it remains unclear whether regeneration or further degeneration occurs [22]. Additionally, significant scuffing can decrease visibility for the surgeon during procedure and can cause misdiagnosis by inexperienced surgeons.

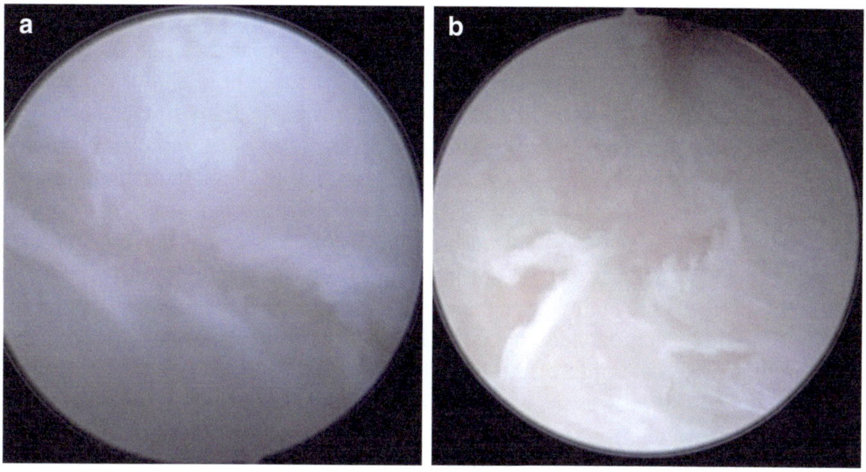

Fig. 11.11 (a) Arthroscopic scuffing and iatrogenic chondromalacia. (b) Arthroscopic scuffing and iatrogenic chondromalacia

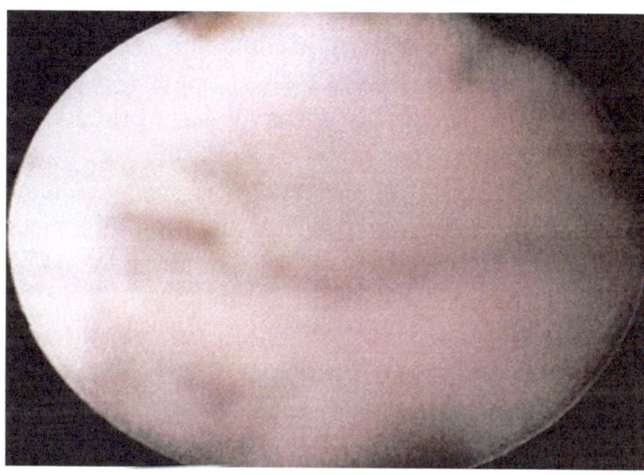

Fig. 11.12 Complete "white out" from fibrous ankylosis

A second complication that can cause disease progression if not handled properly is hemarthrosis leading to fibrous ankylosis ("white out" joint) (Fig. 11.12). Hemarthrosis can be caused by excessive bleeding into the joint space during puncture from tearing of the superficial temporal vessels, from tearing of severely inflamed synovium/retrodiscal tissue upon entrance, and from bleeding of the pterygoid artery during lateral pterygoid myotomy in level IIIb procedures. Although extremely rare, the bleeding can be severe enough to cause termination of the procedure [23]. Typically, pressure and irrigation in addition to some other measures can control bleeding and allow for continuation of the procedure with good visualization of the joint. If hemorrhage is not properly addressed, it will lead to a joint congested with blood. This prolongs healing, increases postoperative discomfort, extends recovery time, and can ultimately lead to fibrous ankylosis.

When hemorrhage inhibits visualization during the procedure, there is a clear protocol to follow. If there is a pointed source, cautery or laser can be used to seal the vessel. If there is not, insufflate the joint with irrigating fluid and/or hyaluronic acid and cover the outflows of the cannulas for 5 min so that sufficient pressure develops to tamponade the bleeding site. If bleeding continues, remove all instruments from the joint and apply direct, external pressure to the preauricular area for an additional 5 min. After 5 min passes, reinsert the instruments and assess the joint. If bleeding still continues, it may be possible to insert a No. 4 catheter balloon through the second portal. Inflate the balloon with normal saline and leave it for 5 min; then deflate and again assess the joint space. Finally, if bleeding still persists, the joint should be approached via open surgery and the area should be packed and any bleeding vessels clamped or cauterized. It is rare in experienced hands to require transition to open surgery as most conservative measures generally work to tamponade bleeding. To avoid fibrous ankylosis in these patients, it is of utmost importance to begin them on a rigorous physical therapy regimen postoperative day 1 and follow them closely throughout the first 6 weeks of healing.

Level IIIb arthroscopy is reserved for the carefully selected patient. It may be beneficial in these situations. The ideal candidate has no signs of active inflammation or primary arthritis and has a Wilkes II or early Wilkes III derangement. This may in fact be there first surgical intervention when the disc displacement is thought to be the primary source of their symptoms. If performed in patients who are late Wilkes III, Wilkes IV, or Wilkes V, have primary inflammatory arthritis, or have active inflammation or joint effusion, the success of the procedure significantly decreases. This is likely the result of persistent inflammation which can cause scarification and adhesions during healing. Therefore, in a patient with active inflammation, it is important to first scope and lavage the joint; then when it is quiescent, if the patient is still symptomatic or closed lock recurs, discopexy can be performed.

Arthroscopic discopexy is performed by first establishing the glenoid fossa and anterior recess portals. Then once inside the anterior recess, the surgeon must identify the disc crease – this is where the disc abuts the lateral pterygoid muscle medially. The surgeon then completes the lateral pterygoid myotomy or anterior release with laser and electrocautery to control bleeding (Fig. 11.13a, b). It is

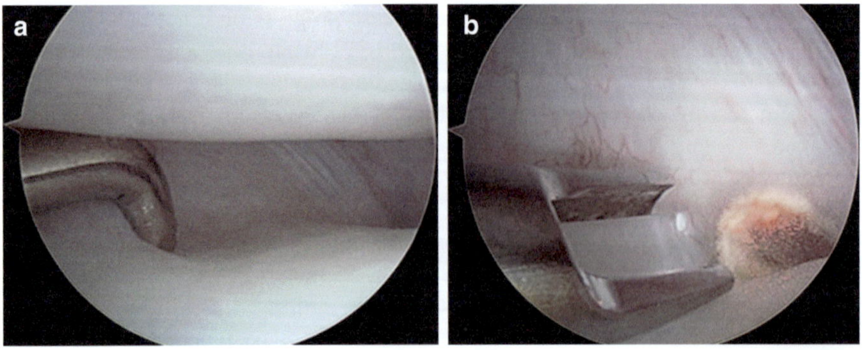

Fig. 11.13 (**a**) Identify the disc crease with a probe. (**b**) Lateral pterygoid myotomy with a laser

important to identify exactly where the disc crease is for two reasons. First, one of the most common complications here can be injury to the disc itself. Second, if the laser is aimed too high into the muscle belly where the vasculature is, this will cause increased bleeding into the joint. Once this is completed, the surgeon brings the scope and instrumentation into the posterior recess to reduce the disc (Fig. 11.14). While the disc is being reduced, two additional smaller ports are obtained. One port is to pass the suture through the disc and the other is to catch the suture (Fig. 11.15). Suture materials have varied from polypropylene suture to wire. Once the suture or wire has been successfully passed through the disc and secured into place, mechanical contracture of the retrodiscal tissue is performed with laser or coblation (Fig. 11.16).

As the disc is the most manipulated anatomical structure in this procedure, one would think it is at risk for injury. However, damage to it is very unlikely when entering the joint space or executing the procedure if the surgeon does not deviate from the standard techniques. The only part of the procedure which violates the disc fibrocartilage itself is during the actual suturing where small perforations into the disc are made with a 20 gauge needle which will heal with time.

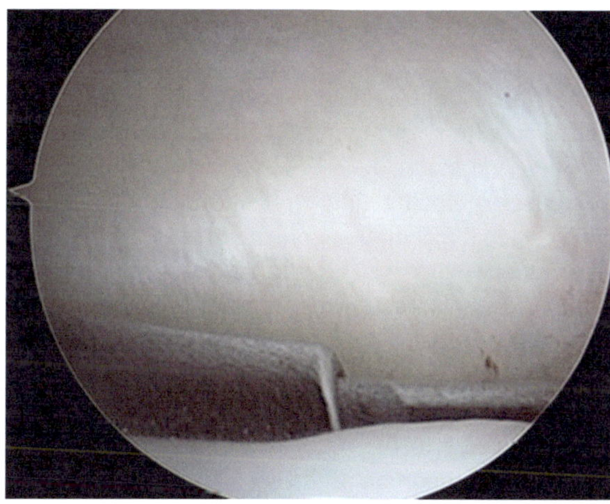

Fig. 11.14 Disc reduction in the posterior recess

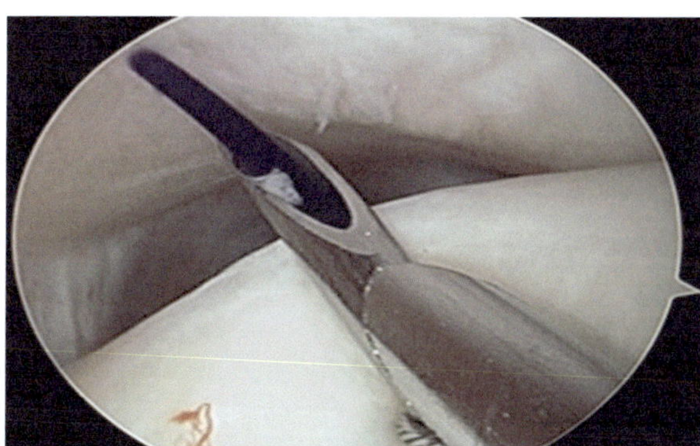

Fig. 11.15 Catching the suture as it is passed through the disc

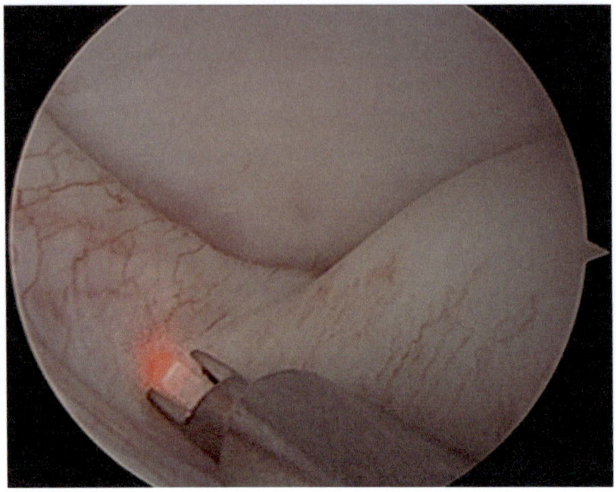

Fig. 11.16 Mechanical contracture of lax retrodiscal tissue with laser

11.2 Open Procedures

11.2.1 Open Discopexy

Although described more than 100 years ago by Annandale, disc repositioning gained popularity following description of the technique and favorable outcomes by McCarty and Farrar in 1979 [24]. Open discopexy can be completed using several techniques including suture plication and the use of anchors and screws although the most ideal technique to plicate the disc remains unclear and outcomes following all techniques appear to be similar. Patient-reported outcomes suggest a success rate of more than 90% in terms of pain, MIO, and function [24–33]. The most ideal indication for this procedure include Wilkes II and early III internal derangement (ID) [34]. It may also be performed on late Wilkes III and IV ID although it is more challenging in part due to the presence of a dysmorphic disc.

After access to the joint is obtained, and the lateral collateral check ligament incised, a small portion of the lax lateral retrodiscal tissue is excised. The disc is then mobilized by releasing its anterior portion through instrumentation and reduced back over the condylar head. A lateral pterygoid myotomy can be performed simultaneously to increase disc mobility although the effect this has on the joint vascularity remains unknown. Following disc mobilization, a posterior and lateral plication is completed with sutures. Discopexy can also be completed with a non-resorbable Mitek®[1] or resorbable JuggerKnot™[2] anchor. When placing an anchor, it is different from suture discopexy in that it employs rigid fixation of the disc to the condylar head. At this point, the anchor drill is used to drill a small pilot hole through the posterior lateral aspect of the condylar head approximately 8 mm from the superior aspect of

[1] ®Depuy Synthes, Raynham, MA.

[2] ™Zimmer Biomet, Jacksonville, FL.

the condyle. The anchor is then inserted and secured in the prepared position through a cleat system. The double-threaded 0/0 non-resorbable suture is passed through the posterior aspect of the disc on both the medial and lateral sides prior to securing it in place. Additional plication of the disc to the retrodiscal tissue and lateral inferior capsule is then completed typically using a smaller suture such as 4/0 or 3/0 Vicryl®[3] or Mersilene®. Once it is secure, the joint is irrigated and the wound is closed.

Potential complications specific to discopexy include the long-term stability of the disc position. Although the immediate postoperative disc position following discopexy appears to be normal in more than 90% of subjects [35], the disc position appears to be less stable with disc displacement reported in many subjects in the long term [31, 36]. Long-term disc stability does not appear to correlate with pain and function [31, 37]. Nevertheless, the potential for subsequent disc displacement with symptoms and the need for a second surgical procedure exist. As with any open joint procedure, discopexy can also result in disc adhesions and progressive degenerative joint disease. The risk can be lessened with attention to technique, meticulous hemostasis, and early joint movement. Initial concerns with the use of the anchor technique revolved around the potential for condylar head resorption as a result of placing the anchor. This appears to be more theoretical than real-based 3-year follow-up data [38].

11.2.2 Open Discectomy with and Without Interpositional Grafting

If the patient has failed all arthroscopic measures and falls into a category Wilkes IV or V, the next surgical step is typically discectomy. The discs are usually dysmorphic and are irreparable. Discectomy involves removing the entire avascular portion of the disc and inflamed retrodiscal tissue. Despite the open surgical approach, it can be very challenging to access all aspects of the disc, especially the medial aspect. The most controversial aspect of performing discectomy is the need for reconstruction and what material to use. The anatomical goal following discectomy is the formation of a pseudo-disc composed of dense collagen. This in theory would serve to provide some load distribution and reduce degenerative changes within the condyle and eminence. This has been routinely observed following discectomy. The purpose of using an interpositional graft is to facilitate the development of the pseudo-disc by placing tissue between the condyle and fossa at the time of surgery.

Patient-reported outcomes after discectomy without replacement have also been reported to be successful in more than a 90% of patients as assessed with pain, MIO, and function [39–47]. Postoperative changes following discectomy typically include progressive degenerative joint disease [39, 42, 48–50]. It remains unclear whether these changes are more severe than those following the use of an interpositional graft. Furthermore, the clinical significance of these changes may be unimportant given the long-term data supporting pain reduction and increase in the MIO and function.

---

[3] ®Ethicon, Johnson and Johnson

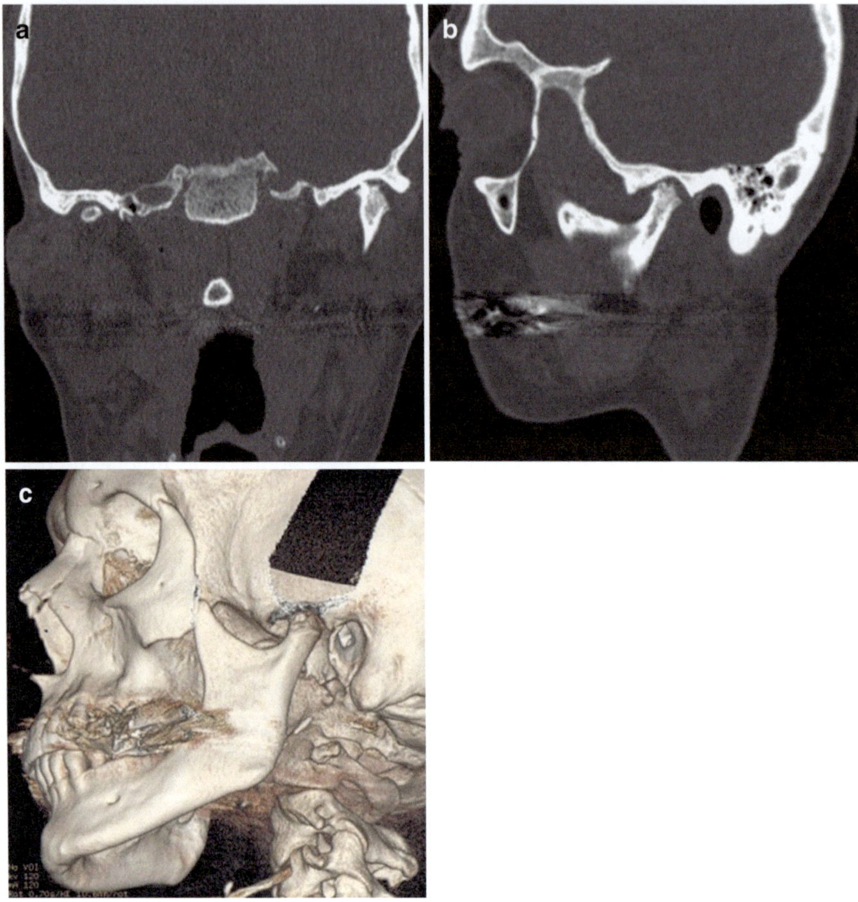

Fig. 11.17 Condylar changes 1 year after discectomy with temporalis flap to left temporomandibular joint. (**a**) Coronal view. (**b**) Sagittal View. (**c**) 3D view

Progression of condylar changes and resorption after discectomy can potentially be delayed or reduced by the placement of an interpositional graft. Interpositional grafting materials include fat, auricular cartilage, full thickness skin, fascia and dermis, temporalis muscle, allogeneic grafts, and temporary Silastic. Each material has its advantages and disadvantages with little scientific evidence to support or refute the material chosen. All have been shown to reduce pain and improve function in a majority of appropriately selected patients. All can be expected to result in radiographic condylar changes consistent with progressive degeneration despite improvement in pain and function (Fig. 11.17a–c).

The potential for iatrogenic degenerative joint disease appears to be greatest following open joint procedures. Although counterintuitive, the development of degenerative joint disease following many varying open joint procedures does not appear to correlate with patient outcomes despite clear radiographic evidence in many patients. This suggests that the inflammatory milieu and disc position/shape and their respective treatment are more important than radiographic features of DJD in predicting patient outcomes. However, the development or progression of degenerative joint disease following discopexy or discectomy with or without replacement does influence the nature of the subsequent surgery should it become necessary.

11.2.3 Total Joint Replacement (TJR)

Indications for total joint replacement include osteoarthritis, ankylosis, failed autogenous grafts or loss of vertical mandibular height secondary to trauma, developmental abnormality, or pathology. Although not mandatory, most patients being considered for TJR should have undergone less invasive surgical procedures initially including arthrocentesis and arthroscopy. Most but not all may also have undergone an open procedure. However, the use of TJR should be considered as the initial open procedure in some patients.

Patient selection is critical as it is with all joint procedures. Multiply-operated patients are at significant risk for worse outcomes as a result of multiple factors [51]. These include the development of peripheral sensitization, central sensitization, neuropathic pain, and maladaptive psychosocial behavior. Therefore, most clinicians recommend only one open surgery prior to considering performing a TJR as this will increase the likelihood of success.

The TJR systems that are currently approved by the Food and Drug Administration (FDA) included both stock and custom devices. They are biocompatible and show good longevity with little wear. The first attempts and partial and total joint replacement in the late 1970s involved the use of materials that lacked the appropriate biocompatibility and wear characteristics. Polytetrafluoroethylene (Teflon), Proplast (Teflon carbon and Teflon aluminum), and Silastic were all used and resulted in catastrophic failures from wear, giant cell reactions, and progressive degenerative changes in the condyle and glenoid fossa. The current TJR systems use the same materials used in total knee and total hip arthroplasties and have undergone extensive laboratory and clinical studies under the auspices of the FDA. An FDA postmarketing surveillance is currently underway to gain further insight into the device performance over time.

Complications specific to TJR are uncommon. Early postoperative infections are uncommon but may present within the first month following surgery. Swelling, fever, suppuration, fistula, and wound breakdown may herald the development of an infection. Meticulous attention to sterility during the procedure including prior irrigation of the external auditory meatus with antibiotic solution, good skin preparation, good draping, minimizing the surgery time, minimizing the number of "try ins" during the procedure, and attention to not contaminating the device or wound with oral flora are crucial. The management of infections remains challenging although protocols to salvage early infections have been reported by Wolford with reasonable success [52]. Delayed infections are more challenging to identify as the signs and symptoms may be more subtle. Delayed infections are most likely from contamination at the time of surgery although hematological seeding from transient bacteremia is also possible. Delayed infections usually involve biofilms that remain resistant to antibiotics. The diagnosis and management of delayed infections requires joint explantation and has been described by Mercuri [53].

As a result of tribo-corrosion, a TJR cannot be expected to last a lifetime, and ultimately this needs to be considered when placing the devices. Young patients are likely to need additional joint replacement, and while this is not considered a complication, the need for additional surgery may result in additional complications. The potential for TJR failure as a result of metal hypersensitivity remains controversial. The very nature of tribo-corrosion ensures that both metal ion release and particulate debris develop after all joint replacement. The particulate debris and a nonspecific immune response to the material seem to correlate with aseptic joint loosening in some patients following total hip arthroplasty and total knee arthroplasty. This has not been identified in TMJ TJR. Metal ion release has been measured in serum following orthopedic and TMJ TJR. Metal ions have been identified in many organs but without any evidence of disease or pathology. Metal ions do have the potential to bind serum proteins to form haptens that can stimulate the immune system resulting in hypersensitivity when tested using patch testing or the leukocyte transforming test (LTT). This seems more common with nickel, cobalt, and chromium which are components of the TMJ TJR condylar head. Routine testing for hypersensitivity to the metal components in orthopedic TJR is not recommended by the manufacturers, FDA, or the American Association of Orthopedic Surgeons despite more than one million implanted devices per year. The development and clinical significance of documented hypersensitivity following TMJ TJR remains unclear, and further research is required before recommendations can be developed to guide best practices.

As with all devices, materials used to manufacture TJR are subject to fatigue and failure. This may result in the loosening or failure of device components. Annual follow-up following TMJ TJR seems prudent to ensure the complications are recognized early and device components replaced as needed.

References

1. Henry CH, Hughes CV, Gerard HC, Hudson AP, Wolford LM. Reactive arthritis: preliminary microbiologic analysis of the human temporomandibular joint. J Oral Maxillofac Surg. 2000;58:1137–42; discussion 43–4.
2. Milam SB, Zardeneta G, Schmitz JP. Oxidative stress and degenerative temporomandibular joint disease: a proposed hypothesis. J Oral Maxillofac Surg. 1998;56:214–23.
3. Dijkgraaf LC, Zardeneta G, Cordewener FW, et al. Crosslinking of fibrinogen and fibronectin by free radicals: a possible initial step in adhesion formation in osteoarthritis of the temporomandibular joint. J Oral Maxillofac Surg. 2003;61:101–11.
4. Sheets Jr DW, Okamoto T, Dijkgraaf LC, Milam SB, Schmitz JP, Zardeneta G. Free radical damage in facsimile synovium: correlation with adhesion formation in osteoarthritic TMJs. J Prosthodont. 2006;15:9–19.

5. Zardeneta G, Milam SB, Lee T, Schmitz JP. Detection and preliminary characterization of matrix metalloproteinase activity in temporomandibular joint lavage fluid. Int J Oral Maxillofac Surg. 1998;27:397–403.
6. Zardeneta G, Milam SB, Schmitz JP. Presence of denatured hemoglobin deposits in diseased temporomandibular joints. J Oral Maxillofac Surg 1997;55:1242–8; discussion
7. Zardeneta G, Milam SB, Schmitz JP. Elution of proteins by continuous temporomandibular joint arthrocentesis. J Oral Maxillofac Surg. 1997;55:709–16; discussion 16–7.
8. Zardeneta G, Milam SB, Schmitz JP. Iron-dependent generation of free radicals: plausible mechanisms in the progressive deterioration of the temporomandibular joint. J Oral Maxillofac Surg. 2000;58:302–8; discussion 9.
9. Bouloux GF. Temporomandibular joint pain and synovial fluid analysis: a review of the literature. J Oral Maxillofac Surg. 2009;67:2497–504.
10. Kaneyama K, Segami N, Nishimura M, Sato J, Fujimura K, Yoshimura H. The ideal lavage volume for removing bradykinin, interleukin-6, and protein from the temporomandibular joint by arthrocentesis. J Oral Maxillofac Surg. 2004;62:657–61.
11. Nitzan DW. Arthrocentesis–incentives for using this minimally invasive approach for temporomandibular disorders. Oral Maxillofac Surg Clin North Am. 2006;18:311–28, vi.
12. McCain JP, Balazs EA, de la Rua H. Preliminary studies on the use of a viscoelastic solution in arthroscopic surgery of the temporomandibular joint. J Oral Maxillofac Surg. 1989;47:1161–8.
13. Stoustrup P, Kristensen KD, Kuseler A, Pedersen TK, Herlin T. Temporomandibular joint steroid injections in patients with juvenile idiopathic arthritis: an observational pilot study on the long-term effect on signs and symptoms. Pediatr Rheumatol Online J. 2015;13:62.
14. Bouloux GF, Chou J, Krishnan D, et al. Is hyaluronic acid or corticosteroid superior to lactated ringer solution in the short-term reduction of temporomandibular joint pain after arthrocentesis? J Oral Maxillofacial Surg. 2017;75:52–62.
15. Bouloux GF, Chou J, Krishnan D, et al. Is hyaluronic acid or corticosteroid superior to lactated ringer solution in the short term for improving function and quality of life after arthrocentesis? J Oral Maxillofacial Surg. 2017;75:63–72.
16. Buckwalter JA, Brown TD. Joint injury, repair, and remodeling: roles in post-traumatic osteoarthritis. Clin Orthop Relat Res. 2004;423:7–16.
17. Meheux CJ, McCulloch PC, Lintner DM, Varner KE, Harris JD. Efficacy of intra-articular platelet-rich plasma injections in knee osteoarthritis: a systematic review. Arthroscopy. 2016;32:495–505.
18. Comert Kılic S, Gungormus M, Sumbullu MA. Is arthrocentesis plus platelet-rich plasma superior to arthrocentesis alone in the treatment of temporomandibular joint osteoarthritis? A randomized clinical trial. J Oral Maxillofac Surg. 2015;73:1473–83.
19. Goss AN, Bosanquet AG. Temporomandibular joint arthroscopy. J Oral Maxillofac Surg. 1986;44:614–7.
20. Holmlund A, Hellsing G. Arthroscopy of the temporomandibular joint. An autopsy study. Int J Oral Surg. 1985;14:169–75.
21. Westesson PL, Eriksson L, Liedberg J. The risk of damage to facial nerve, superficial temporal vessels, disk, and articular surfaces during arthroscopic examination of the temporomandibular joint. Oral Surg Oral Med Oral Pathol. 1986;62:124–7.
22. Weiss C, Mirow S. An ultrastructural study of osteoarthritis changes in the articular cartilage of human knees. J Bone Joint Surg Am. 1972;54:954–72.
23. McCain JP, de la Rua H, LeBlanc WG. Puncture technique and portals of entry for diagnostic and operative arthroscopy of the temporomandibular joint. Arthroscopy. 1991;7:221–32.
24. McCarty WL, Farrar WB. Surgery for internal derangements of the temporomandibular joint. J Prosthet Dent. 1979;42:191–6.
25. Mercuri LG, Campbell RL, Shamaskin RG. Intra-articular meniscus dysfunction surgery. A preliminary report. Oral Surg Oral Med Oral Pathol. 1982;54:613–21.
26. Hall MB. Meniscoplasty of the displaced temporomandibular joint meniscus without violating the inferior joint space. J Oral Maxillofac Surg. 1984;42:788–92.

27. Walker RV, Kalamchi S. A surgical technique for management of internal derangement of the temporomandibular joint. J Oral Maxillofac Surg. 1987;45:299–305.
28. Kerstens HC, Tuinzing DB, van der Kwast WA. Eminectomy and discoplasty for correction of the displaced temporomandibular joint disc. J Oral Maxillofac Surg. 1989;47:150–4.
29. Dolwick MF, Nitzan DW. The role of Disc-repositioning surgery for internal derangements of the temporomandibular joint. Oral Maxillofac Surg Clin North Am. 1994;6:271.
30. Bays R. Temporomandibular joint disc preservation. Atlas Oral Maxillofac Surg Clin North Am. 1996;4:33.
31. Montgomery MT, Gordon SM, Van Sickels JE, Harms SE. Changes in signs and symptoms following temporomandibular joint disc repositioning surgery. J Oral Maxillofac Surg. 1992;50:320–8.
32. Piper M. Microscopic disc preservation surgery of the temporomandibular joint. Oral Maxfac Surg Clin North Am. 1989;1:279.
33. Marciani RD, Ziegler RC. Temporomandibular joint surgery: a review of fifty-one operations. Oral Surg Oral Med Oral Pathol. 1983;56:472–6.
34. Mehra P, Wolford LM. The Mitek mini anchor for TMJ disc repositioning: surgical technique and results. Int J Oral Maxillofac Surg. 2001;30:497–503.
35. Zhang S, Liu X, Yang X, et al. Temporomandibular joint disc repositioning using bone anchors: an immediate post surgical evaluation by magnetic resonance imaging. BMC Musculoskelet Disord. 2010;11:262.
36. Westesson PL, Cohen JM, Tallents RH. Magnetic resonance imaging of temporomandibular joint after surgical treatment of internal derangement. Oral Surg Oral Med Oral Pathol. 1991;71:407–11.
37. Abramowicz S, Dolwick MF. 20-year follow-up study of disc repositioning surgery for temporomandibular joint internal derangement. J Oral Maxillofac Surg. 2010;68:239–42.
38. Fields RT, Jr, Wolford LM. The osseointegration of Mitek mini anchors in the mandibular condyle. J Oral Maxillofac Surg. 2001;59:1402–6; discussion 7.
39. Eriksson L, Westesson PL. Long-term evaluation of meniscectomy of the temporomandibular joint. J Oral Maxillofac Surg. 1985;43:263–9.
40. Silver CM. Long-term results of meniscectomy of the temporomandibular joint. Cranio. 1984;3:46–57.
41. Tolvanen M, Oikarinen VJ, Wolf J. A 30-year follow-up study of temporomandibular joint meniscectomies: a report on five patients. Br J Oral Maxillofac Surg. 1988;26:311–6.
42. Gundlach KK. Long-term results following surgical treatment of internal derangement of the temporomandibular joint. J Craniomaxillofac Surg. 1990;18:206–9.
43. Hall DH. The role of discectomy for treating internal derangements of the temporomandibular joint. Oral Maxfac Surg Clin North Am. 1994;6:287.
44. Bjornland T, Larheim TA. Discectomy of the temporomandibular joint: 3-year follow-up as a predictor of the 10-year outcome. J Oral Maxillofac Surg. 2003;61:55–60.
45. McKenna SJ. Discectomy for the treatment of internal derangements of the temporomandibular joint. J Oral Maxillofac Surg. 2001;59:1051–6.
46. Nyberg J, Adell R, Svensson B. Temporomandibular joint discectomy for treatment of unilateral internal derangements–a 5 year follow-up evaluation. Int J Oral Maxillofac Surg. 2004;33:8–12.
47. Miloro M, Henriksen B. Discectomy as the primary surgical option for internal derangement of the temporomandibular joint. J Oral Maxillofac Surg. 2010;68:782–9.
48. Brown WA. Internal derangement of the temporomandibular joint: review of 214 patients following meniscectomy. Can J Surg. 1980;23:30–2.
49. Holmlund AB, Gynther G, Axelsson S. Diskectomy in treatment of internal derangement of the temporomandibular joint. Follow-up at 1, 3, and 5 years. Oral Surg Oral Med Oral Pathol. 1993;76:266–71.
50. Agerberg G, Lundberg M. Changes in the temporomandibular joint after surgical treatment. A radiologic follow-up study. Oral Surg Oral Med Oral Pathol. 1971;32:865–75.

51. Mercuri LG. Subjective and objective outcomes in patients reconstructed with a custom-fitted alloplastic temporomandibular joint prosthesis. J Oral Maxillofac Surg. 1999;57:1427–30.
52. Wolford LM, Rodrigues DB, McPhillips A. Management of the infected temporomandibular joint total joint prosthesis. J Oral Maxillofac Surg. 2010;68:2810–23.
53. Mercuri LG. Avoiding and managing temporomandibular joint total joint replacement surgical site infections. J Oral Maxillofac Surg. 2012;70:2280–9.

MIX
Papier aus verantwortungsvollen Quellen
Paper from responsible sources
FSC® C105338
FSC
www.fsc.org

If you have any concerns about our products,
you can contact us on
ProductSafety@springernature.com

In case Publisher is established outside the EU,
the EU authorized representative is:
Springer Nature Customer Service Center GmbH
Europaplatz 3, 69115 Heidelberg, Germany

Printed by Libri Plureos GmbH
in Hamburg, Germany